WORKING KNIGHTS

This is a book about medicine. It contains the personal opinions and observations of the author, formed over many years in the practice of medicine. This work is intended strictly for entertainment purposes only. It is not a textbook or treatment guideline and should not be used as such. Any reader who believes that they have a medical problem should consult a physician, rather than using the author's rambling sarcasm as any sort of medical advice.

Some of the observations and stories presented here concern real incidents. All names have been changed, or deleted entirely, to protect individual identity.

Cover art provided by Ray Keys, of The Weekly's. (www.theweeklys.com).

Inside art provided by Samuel Edwin Leap, future cartoonist and illustrator, age 9.

www.edwinleap.com
2004

WORKING KNIGHTS

K. EDWIN LEAP II

Acknowledgments

I would like to thank many people for their assistance with this book. Since the lion's share of words on these pages were first printed in Emergency Medicine News, a publication of Lippincott, Williams and Wilkins, I owe a great debt to Lisa Hoffman, editor of EMN. She has given me a wonderful opportunity by allowing me to write a monthly column for a national audience, and by letting me write about so many different things that touch on the specialty of emergency medicine.

Thanks also to Tom Inman, retired editorial page editor of the Greenville News, who gave me my first break in writing by giving me a regular column in that wonderful newspaper. His wisdom about writing continues to guide me, as we meet over the South's finest Fried Chicken at the Walhalla Steak House.

Further thanks are due to Mary Beth Padgett, current editorial page editor of the Greenville News, who continues to let me to write for the paper twice a month and who graciously tolerates my lack of focus, as my columns range from politics to family, from prescriptions drugs to rattlesnakes.

A few of these pieces were first printed in Physician Magazine, a publication of Focus on the Family that is no longer in production. I'd like to thank Focus on the Family for the privilege of writing for Physician, and especially Scott DeNicola, editor of Physician, for his encouragement and guidance.

I also need to thank my partners in Blue Ridge Emergency Physicians and all my dear friends and co-workers at Oconee Memorial Hospital. They have supported my efforts and we have shared so many great stories, so many sorrows, so much laughter and all those long, exhausting nights down the years.

Most important, I want to thank my wife, Jan, for understanding my need to write. Her constant love and praise, as well as her wise editorial guidance, have kept me on the right path. When she says I have written something well, I know that I've nailed it. When her lip turns up in a smile at something funny I have written, I know that it will get laughs. And when she tells that my sentences are cumbersome and plagued by commas, I know it's time to get back to the computer. Her technical abilities allowed the manuscript to be prepared, since our computer despises me, but responds to her every touch.

Even as the weeds around our house grow taller and the dogs remain flea-ridden, she allows me to sit in our loft and write, because she knows that it is important to me. I could have married other women. I could not have loved any as much as I love my bride. Proverbs 31:29 says, "Many women do noble things, but you surpass them all".

Further thanks to Samuel, Seth, Elijah and Elysa, for understanding when I write. My children still smile when they see my face in the newspaper or in copies of Emergency Medicine News. And they know that even though I may be typing madly, it won't be long until I'm back on the trampoline with them at the end of the session or the end of the day. You four are the best and you constantly inspire me. I love you all.

Thanks to God for all of you and for all the things in life to write about.

Table of Contents

Preface ix
A Brief Glossary of Terms for the Non-Medical xiii
The Golden Rule Revisited 1
Watching in the Night 4
Flu Season Fun 7
Jack's Place 9
A Little Pat on the Back 12
Creatures of the Night 16
Ambiguity 17
Aliens in Our Midst 19
An Old Woman's Memories 23
Compassion has a Price 25
Crazy is as Crazy Does 27
Barbarians are Alive and Well 30
Even Doctors Get Sick 32
The Big Possums Walk the Night 35
A Little Summer Fun 37
The Voices in My Head 39
Making Sense of Loss 43
Oh to be Obsolete 45
Rural Practice 47
The Blessed Mundane 50
Beautiful Girl 52
Time and Children 53
DUI—Driving Un-Impeded 56
Breath Shepherd 59
Quality of Life 62
A Prayer For Us 64
Grandpa's Hands 65
The Worst Lie is the One You Tell Yourself 68
Hope for my Child's Disease 74

The Mysteries of the Night 78
Betrayed by my Slacks 82
HIPAA: Madness Legislated 84
Why Emergency Departments Close 87
I Want to Eat Your Head 90
Angelic Visitations 94
Saving Our Own Lives 97
Vulnerability of a Father 100
Making a House Call 104
It's Better Incognito 106
Prescription for Hypocrisy 108
Getting Stoned (in the Kidney) 113
Did You Hear the One About the Lawyer? 115
The Real Power of Medicine 117
Everyone is Fighting a Great Battle 119
Coping with My Fear of the Night 122
What do you call an Emergency Physician? 124
The Gifts of the Dead 126
Doing Less is More 129
Important Discharge Instructions 131
A Jealous Mistress 136
Lost in the Wilderness of the Mind 139
Trailer Trash 141
Bobby, Jimmy and the big, honkin' snake 144
Fear 147
Crosses 149
The White Knights of Medicine 151
Author Biography 155

Preface

I never cared much for alcohol. I never used drugs. I have smoked one or two cigars, but no cigarettes. I have been enthralled by one woman my entire adult life. But I have an addiction and it's to stories and the books where they are found. I walk through bookstores like some people linger before jewelry cases. I buy far too many books, because borrowing them just isn't enough. I have always been this way. I have always needed more stories, more words, more insights. Looking back, I have been reading poetry and novels and everything else since I can remember. And the only pain I feel in the presence of books is that there are so many that I will never read in this life.

I wanted to be a writer for a while, when I was young. I started my education in journalism. But in an odd twist, I fell into medicine. Now, fourteen years after graduating from medical school, I see how perfect it was. Because medicine allowed me into some of the most profound stories imaginable and let me insert myself in them as a character, major and minor.

A few years ago the stories began to erupt onto paper, as newspaper columns on the op-ed page of the Greenville News, where they continue to appear. I told the stories of people I had seen and tried to make connections to their situations or lives that readers could relate to. Much of what they contained came from my practice of medicine, which is that of working in a rural emergency department (some of us still call it an emergency room). But my beliefs, views and opinions, my anger and my humor, were deeply influenced by my new experience of fatherhood. Suddenly most of the things that affected me or moved me could be related to my wife and children, even if they originated in a hospital trauma bay. Through fatherhood, I learned about the depth of love that a man can feel and about the fears that haunt us most in this fragile life. Through fatherhood, my bond with my patients, my interest in their stories became more profound than ever.

But even as I understood the human experience better, my progressive years in medicine also made me see some inescapable truths. Over time, my writing began to take on a different edge. It became a voice of frustration with the medical system, an expression of my anger at being used by government and by an annoying minority of my patients. I began writing for a professional magazine called Emergency Medicine News. There, I was writing for physicians and other health care workers. There, I could vent all of the frustration of our jobs. I am a physician advocate, in an age in which it was only fashionable to be a patient advocate. I write about regulations and rules, drug abusers and violence, confusing medical complaints and obnoxious doctors. In time, my readers began to ask me for copies and collections of my columns. The idea stewed in my mind.

In time, I was printed in Physician Magazine, a Christian magazine for the medical community, Physician allowed me to galvanize my faith with my view of people. There I could speak about God and man without fear of alienation, without fear that I would be considered preachy. It was truly a blessing for my writing, appearing as everything had when the time was just right.

So here are many of my columns. Reprinted, edited a little, sometimes re-titled. They come mostly from Emergency Medicine News, as well as few from the Greenville News and Physician Magazine. A few have never been published until now. They cross a lot of boundaries. Some are about the pain I see in the lives of the patients and staff in the emergency room. Some are about the pain I feel when I take care of very difficult people. In these re-incarnated columns I may seem overly sentimental or overly vain. I may seem as if I want to save the world and then seem as if I just wish everyone would leave me alone. If one of them annoys you, ignore it and read another. A number of these were written for physicians. These are frustrating days in medicine. Admittedly, we have good jobs and we whine too much. But much of what we complain about is legitimate and reflects unfortunate trends in culture and government. So when I write to my brothers and sisters in medicine, I'm writing to encourage and to galvanize the opinions of physicians who have been told not to speak what they feel about politics, but to speak with the sterile voices of a profession populated by too many sheep.

But even if have written a great deal for physicians, the same frustrations and wonders apply to everyone who works in emergency care or in health care in general. So much of what I have to say applies to nurses, paramedics, administrators, risk-managers and all the rest. We all face the same struggles from slightly different angles.

But whatever I write and whatever you read, it's the truth as I see it, with no apology. So here is a look into medicine, into patients, into rules and regulations. Here are my honest attempts to make available all the trouble, all the delight and all the lunacy. And here, in these columns that wander from topic to topic like a Saturday night drunk is the fusion of my loves for God, for family, for all the delightful fruitcakes of the world, for my chosen profession and for the holiness and power of words. Thank you for reading.

(A word about the title: Working Knights derives from the fact that I do, in fact, work nights quite a lot. But the wordplay on nights has to do with the first column I wrote for Emergency Medicine News, entitled White Knights of Medicine. It had the delightful effect of encouraging many emergency physicians and of speaking some truths about the specialty that they had felt were unacceptable to say out loud. It was the column that launched my regular column in Emergency Medicine News. That particular column occupies the last place in this book.)

A Brief Glossary of Terms for the Non-Medical

Medicine is full of odd terms and acronyms. I have kept them to a minimum. But here are a few:

ACEP: American College of Emergency Physicians. This is one of two principal specialty organizations in emergency medicine, the other being the AAEM - American Academy of Emergency Medicine.

ABEM: American Board of Emergency Medicine. This is the organization that confers board certification on emergency physicians, along with the ABOEM - American Board of Osteopathic Emergency Medicine.

ED/ER: Emergency Department/Emergency Room. These acronyms are used interchangeably. Some physicians feel that ED more accurately reflects the fact that ours is a real specialty, not just a job done by anyone standing in the appropriate room at the right time.

EMS: Emergency Medical Services. That is paramedics and others who care for patients before they arrive at the hospital.

EMTALA: Emergency Medical Treatment and Active Labor Act. This law ensures that everyone is seen in the emergency department regardless of ability to pay. That you can bill the patient after giving them care, but you can not ask for money up front.

HIPAA: Health Insurance Portability and Accountability Act. This law exists to help you keep your insurance when changing jobs. It also attempts to ensure the privacy of medical records.

ICU/PICU: Intensive Care Unit or Pediatric Intensive Care Unit

IOM: Institute of Medicine. This quasi-governmental think tank examines problems facing medicine and tries to propose solutions.

JCAHO: Joint Commission for the Accreditation of Hospital Organizations. This organization certifies hospitals and outpatient areas as safe and up-to-date. It establishes many rules for the conduct of patient care.

MVA: A motor vehicle accident

Pain Scale: A scale usually numbered one through ten or showing smiling and frowning faces for children. It is currently used to assess degree of pain in patients, as well as the adequacy (or inadequacy) of the treatment they are receiving for pain.

SIDS: Sudden Infant Death Syndrome

Residency: The training a physician receives after medical school. It may last three or four years (as in emergency medicine) or as long as six or seven years for certain surgical specialties. Fellowships tack on extra time beyond that. Internship, in common usage, generally means the first year of a residency.

The Golden Rule Revisited

They lie there, breathing heavy gasps, contracted into a fetal position. Ironic, that they should live 80 or 90 years, then return to the posture of their childhood. But they do. Sometimes their voices are mumbles and whispers like those of infants or toddlers. I have seen them, unaware of anything for decades, crying out for parents long since passed away. I recall one who had begun to sleep excessively and told her daughter that a little girl slept with her each night. I don't know what she saw. Maybe an infant she lost, or a sibling, cousin or friend from years long gone. But I do know what I see when I stand by the bedside of the infirm aged. Though their bodies are skin covered sticks and their minds an inescapable labyrinth, I see something surprising. I see something beautiful and horrible, hopeful and hopeless. What I see is my children, long after I leave them, as they end their days.

This vision comes to me sometimes when I stand by the bedside of a patient and look over the ancient form that lies before me, barely aware of anything. Usually the feeling comes in those times when I am weary and frustrated from making too many decisions too fast, in the middle of the night. Into the midst of this comes a patient from a local nursing home, sent for reasons I can seldom discern. I walk into the room and roll my cynical eyes at the nurse. She hands me the minimal data sent with the patient and I begin the detective work. And just when I'm most annoyed, just when I want to do nothing and send them back, I look at them. And then I touch them. And then, as I imagine my four little children, tears well up and I see the error of my thoughts. For one day it may be. One day, my little boys and girl, still young enough to kiss me and think me heroic, may lie before another cynical doctor, in the middle of the night of their dementia and need care. More than medicine, they will need compassion. They will need for someone to have the insight to look at them and say, "Here was once a child, cherished and loved, who played games in the nursery with his mother and father. Here was a child who put teeth under pillows, and loved bedtime stories, crayons and stuffed animals. Here was a treasure of love to a man and a woman long gone. How can I honor them? By treating their child with love and gentility. By seeing that their child has come full circle to infancy once more and will soon be born once more into forever."

This vision is frightful because I will not be there to comfort them, or to say, "I am here" when they call out, unless God grants me the gift of speaking across forever. It is painful because I will not be there to serve them as I did in life and see that they are treated as what they are: unique and wonderful, made in the image of the Creator and of their mother and me. It is terrible because our society treats the aged as worse than a burden; it treats them as tragedies of time. It seems hopeless because when they contract and lie motionless, no one will touch them with the love I have for them, or know the history of their scars, visible and invisible. I am the walking library of their lives and I will be unavailable. All I can do is ask, while I live, for God's mercy on them as they grow older.

And yet, the image has beauty and hope as well. Because, if I see my children as aged and infirm, I can dream that their lives were long and rich. I can dream that they filled their lucid years with greatness and love; that they knew God and served him well and were persons of honor and gentility. I can imagine that even if they live in their shadow land alone, somewhere children and grandchildren, even great grandchildren thrive. I can hope that their heirs come to see them and care and harass the staff of the nursing home to treat Grandpa or Grandma better. I can hope that they dare not allow my boys to suffer, but that they hold no illusions about physical immortality and will let them come to their mother and me when the time arrives. And best, I can know that their age and illness will only bring the day of that reunion closer.

My career as a physician has taught me something very important about dealing with the sick and injured, whether young or old. It has taught me that the Golden Rule can also be stated this way: "Do unto others as you would have others do unto your children." I think that this is a powerful way to improve our interactions with others, not just in medicine, but in every action of our lives. And it is certainly a unique way to view our treatment of the elderly. For one day all our children will be old. And only if this lesson has been applied will they be treated with anything approaching the love that only we, their parents, hope for them to always have.

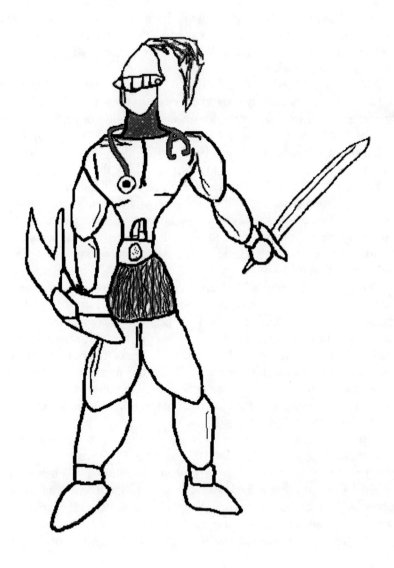

Watching in the Night

There are things I love about the night. I love the stillness and the way it feels on clear southern nights when I have the sensation I am driving among the moon and stars on the way to work. I love the cooler air, the silence, the mystery. People who work only in the daytime miss a lot. Night can be magnificent.

I don't like leaving my family when sleep has enveloped the children. I hate the way it feels to cover them with a blanket, close the door and go out into the world, knowing that I will not be there if they are sick or in danger. I hate kissing my wife goodbye when she is curled up in her robe, reading a book in our dimly lit living room. It seems hateful and blasphemous to leave such holy things behind.

But that's what I do; I work at night. One of the problems with emergency medicine, and with medicine in general, is that it never stops. Medicine is a ship and there's always an officer of the watch. About twelve nights every month, I'm that officer. I accept that duty because it is a necessity. Besides, there are things about practicing at night that I find pleasant.

Once when I couldn't sleep, I thought back on my medical education and practice and calculated how much of my life had been spent working at night. I've been in practice eleven years. I spent three years in residency, two clinical years in medical school and two academic. But I'll discount those academic years. In spite of late night study sessions, they don't compare to making life-altering decisions in the middle of the night. So the tally comes to some sixteen years in which I have been attempting to live, function and treat patients after the sun has gone below the horizon.

Sometimes I feel a deep ache as my body tries to convince me to sleep those nights when I'm awake. Someday I may have to. But for now I'll stay the course. I have four small children. When I work nights, I can put them to bed before work, see them and send them to school in the morning after work, sleep a bit, then have all evening with them again when they return home. And because I'm willing to work so many nights, I work less each month than most of my partners. My free time with my wife and children is luxurious. I can't throw that away just to work when the sun is warm.

But there's more. I enjoy the night because medicine at night is an adventure. I know that ideally it should be the same as in the day. But I'm not nocturnal by nature. I wasn't meant to be up all night. I do it, but somehow it's wrong. My mind and body aren't at peak performance. That means that nights require special vigilance. Dangerous conditions more easily sneak up on me. And third shift requires a certain insight into the human condition. People act differently between sunset and sunrise.

I've learned through the years that people come to emergency rooms for many reasons at night, but one of the most important ones is fear, pure and simple. As children we learn to fear the night. It's a time of uncertainty. Our ancestors embodied their fears in imaginary monsters, like vampires, witches and werewolves. Something within them was afraid of what they could not see or express. I've worked enough nights to know another reason for that basic human fear. There are, in fact, things out at night that aren't there in the day. Predators, two legged and four, stalk the darkness. Or maybe we learned to fear the night because we weren't always confident that morning would come. Maybe we still wonder the same thing.

Regardless of the source of the fear, patients present with difficult complaints like vague chest pain, numbness, swollen body parts that aren't swollen and many others. Often these bizarre complaints are just the anxiety or loneliness of night. I'm at a point in my practice where I don't attempt to solve all of these puzzles. Instead I often do a minimal work-up to rule out dangerous problems. Then I reassure. Reassurance is a skill vital to the night doctor. "You aren't having a heart attack", "Your baby has a fever, but is just fine", "It's OK that your child ate a piece of deodorant."

Of course bad things sometimes happen at night. I take pride in being available for those times too. People have horrible car wrecks. Drunks shoot and stab one another. Beloved infants die of SIDS. During those times, it is the job of the night doctor to be the one "on the wall"; there to intervene and try and save a life which, not so many years ago, would have been lost because there wasn't much health care

5

available after hours. I've found that this is a lonely job. When I was a resident, in a teaching hospital, there was always another doctor to bail me out of tough spots. Always someone to ask a question. Always someone else to go with me when I had to say, "I'm so sorry, but your wife died." In my community hospital, in my medium sized emergency room, I'm the lone ranger at night.

Like so many things in my life, night shift has become a part of who I am: 'the night doctor, the vampire'. I don't always like the fatigue or the uncertainty. But I love the unique character of the night and its citizens. The night holds secret pleasures for everyone, but especially for doctors. We get to see all of its terror and beauty, and can participate in making it less terrible for everyone else. No matter how tired I get, that fact keeps me coming back each night.

Flu Season Fun

In medical school I thought it was cool to wear my scrub shirt in public. After all people would think I was a doctor. Now I avoid it for the same reason. I was reminded of this when I stepped out of my car one March evening at the hospital where I work. I was immediately identified as a physician and verbally accosted by the family of a patient. "I can't believe how long it's taking! My sister is hurting and someone needs to see her!" The parking lot was overflowing, so I knew the waiting room was as well. I tried my best to explain the problems of patient volume, room availability and staffing. It was typical of the month of March and part of the month of April. It was, and is, a difficulty felt all across the nation.

My fellow health care providers all over South Carolina have been struggling for months under what seems like an infinite number of patients, while working in facilities with finite staff and space. Here are only a few of the reasons: Influenza hit us a little late this year; there have been large numbers of patients with pneumonia and severe intestinal viruses, especially the elderly, who required admission; and there are simply more people in the state (sunny skies and mild winters bring increased populations).

Consequently, patients in emergency departments have been waiting two to ten hour to be seen. Many who have required admission have been spending the night in the emergency department due to lack of beds. The overwhelming majority of patients and families have been wonderfully tolerant and understanding. However, as with anything, it only takes a few angry outbursts to make things difficult.

We in health care know that it is tiresome to wait. But we can't stop the numbers any more than we can build new hospitals or hire more nurses overnight. And we are powerless to make people turn around and go home. Besides, it would be dangerous to do so. Research has suggested that significant numbers of people who leave an emergency department before being evaluated have a serious illness. Simply put, some people are simply too sick to stay for long in the waiting room.

In the midst of the chaos, fuses have been short among patients, families and health care workers. As professionals, it is our duty to

7

remember that people sometimes act unpleasant when they are frightened or ill. This is human nature. But health care providers are people too. We want to be treated with respect and without rage. We don't move faster when cursed, insulted or glared at. We simply want people to follow a very old rule that most are familiar with: "Do unto others as you would have others do unto you."

In America, we love convenience and speed. This is the reason that fast food is so popular. But hospitals, for all their talk about quality assurance, for all their corporate efficiency schemes, can't function like fast food. In a restaurant, it's first come, first served. In an emergency department, some patrons are always more seriously ill than others. Some, in fact, seem to arrive at our door just as the door to the after-life opens before them. So, we allocate resources to the sickest first, regardless of when they arrive. Among those resources are the time that doctors, nurses etc. spend with patients and the physical space that those patients occupy.

Those who waited patiently for care, or rooms, deserve the thanks of all health care providers involved. Those who fought the fight in these frantic months, physicians, nurses, paramedics, respiratory therapists, lab and x-ray technicians, dietitians, housekeeping personnel, etc., should be congratulated for their perseverance and professionalism.

Last night at work I saw a fax from our regional referral center that said they actually had beds and could accept critical transfers. I've had two easy nights in a row. Oh bliss! Maybe things are going to slow down a bit. But even if it doesn't, we'll all keep trying to provide compassionate, effective and expedient care. We simply hope everyone who visits our facility on busy days or nights realizes this.

Jack's Place

I drove past Jack's Place not long ago. I should say, I drove past the lot where Jack's Place used to be. Of course, you wouldn't know anything about Jack's. It was a road-side bar, with walls a stiff wind could take down. It was the kind of bar that you wouldn't go into unless you were suicidal, homicidal or extremely well armed. It's door was always open; literally. The cars and motorcycles that parked outside were usually dusty and worn, just like their drivers. It was a place to go after working a long day of construction in the South Carolina heat. Or when you needed a cold one after evading the state trooper in a high-speed chase. It was a place to go on Saturday night to prove yourself. I suspect it was a reasonable place to go if you wanted anything illegal or immoral. You understand. It was what we in the South call a landmark.

I had always known where Jack's place was. It was across the road from a "fish camp". For those in other geographic areas, a fish camp has nothing to do with camping and precious little to do with fish. The only real connection to fish is that it's the location where former aquatic creatures like fish and shrimp are solidly encased in batter and dropped into the deep fryer. I know my coronary arteries hate me, but boy it was good. One of our nurses worked at the fish camp as a teen. "Those Church of God ladies who run it keep it spotless! You could eat off of the floor!" I wouldn't doubt it.

On the other hand, a lot of people found the floor at Jack's, but I suspect very few ate off of it. It was a stark contrast from the fish camp and it's church ladies. Jack's was a hard place, for hard men and women. I know because I saw a patient from Jack's once. He didn't have much to say, considering the tidy hole in his chest, just next to his upper sternum. I never understood quite how it happened. It was irrelevant. At Jack's place, outside a dim, dirty bar, he took a knife in the chest.

I opened that chest, but I knew what the outcome would be. He had come some fifteen miles by ambulance, over country roads, with his blood pooling in his chest. He had left the pain of this life somewhere along the way. Of course, he didn't bleed much in the parking lot at

Jack's. So maybe his soul didn't leave until I opened him up and looked down into the pool of red that had kept him alive before that evening. Maybe his soul left through the slice in his aorta, just above his heart and escaped when the rib spreaders popped and cracked across him. Maybe.

Even as his life was over, that evening still sparked and crackled with danger. I thought my own life might also be shortened when I told his brother what happened. He punched the conference room door so hard that the police came running, thinking it was a gun shot. Furious for revenge he stormed out, ready to multiply pain. I don't know if he accomplished his goal. I do known that my patient's killer went to prison. One imprisoned above ground, one below. A heavy price for a stop at Jack's Place. A heavy price for anger and recklessness.

And in the midst of it all, it became part of my world. By virtue of my profession, I was pulled into the world of Jack's Place. I became a player in a mad, violent act in a gravel parking lot near Salem, South Carolina. I never had a drink there. I never knew victim or killer. But I became a part of it all when that good ole' boy came to me and I looked inside his body and knew he was finished. I became a part of it all, an indelible memory for others and for me when I told a huge, angry man that his brother had been murdered: when I told his elderly parents he had been murdered. In the process I became more entrenched, more solidly planted in this place that's now my home.

I didn't grow up in these little country towns and communities. But now I'm part of the story, part of the local history. I'm anchored by the tales I know; many of which include me at some point, frequently in the final chapter. I know the good people, pastors and businessmen, laborers and students, mothers and fathers and children. And I know the drug abusers and alcoholics. I know the criminals, wife-beaters and child-abusers. Sometimes I feel like I'm the doctor for the local underworld. A few years of evenings and nights will do that. I've supplied tons of narcotics to people who lie about their pain then sell them on the street. I know that I have cared for men and women wanted for terrible crimes committed locally or in other states. And in the process, I've become part of their legends, however epic or brief.

Likewise they, with their slashed necks and broken arms, bullet holes and beaten faces, have baptized me in their blood and sucked me into lives I didn't want any part of. They have become a part of me.

So it all came back when I drove past Jack's Place. An image of a man with a hole in his chest. My own constructed image of the struggle in the doorway, the struggle by the parked cars. The man down on one knee, clutching his chest, feeling his soul slip out by degrees. I imagined the crowd of people, the police car and ambulance. I wonder if he knew and what he was thinking when the darkness came down. I imagined it all up to the point when I entered the story and actually recall it.

In the field where Jack's used to be, there is now a yard with determined grass growing through the red clay. Even the building is gone, with not so much as the customary pile of rubble to mark it. It isn't a landmark anymore. A trailer with a nice, large porch sits back from the road. I hope there are children there. I think it's nice when kids laugh and play in a place where a man lost his life. Like children running on the grass at Gettysburg or Ypres. It hallows the ground a little. Maybe it gives the dead some solace.

But as for me, that piece of land, that stretch of road will always remind me of his blood. It will always bring back the story of the fight, the knife, the mortal wound. And I don't mind. It may be that in 50 years, I'll be the only one who remembers. I'll accept my role as a walking archive. It's all part of the package we get as physicians. Connections to places and the stories of the people who live and die in them.

A Little Pat on the Back

We physicians spend our careers telling people what's wrong with them. We try to fix the problems and often do. But the process begins with the flaw. It begins with the pain, the fear, the weakness, the sickness. Our job is to tell people the manner in which their bodies or minds are failing, either temporarily or permanently.

But one day I thought to myself how wonderful it would be if we all had someone who would tell us what was right about us. Someone to tell us that we were alright. There isn't much of that in the world. Imagine if you could wake up feeling terrible and go down the street to the office of someone who would simply sit down and tell you everything wonderful about yourself. And not just the self-evident things: not just, "you're very successful", but the little things, the things you hope, but fear to admit. Things like, "You are strong. You are kind. You look very young. You are wise. You may feel like you aren't smart sometimes, but you really are. You have a hidden talent that you haven't discovered, but you will. Your children think that you are a hero. Your wife isn't lying when she says you're irresistible." I'd be there every day. Because we high achieving doctor types have spent our lives working toward our goals, prodded less by our strengths than by our weaknesses (or perceptions of them). It began decades ago. And it hasn't stopped yet.

I can't address all of the personal ghosts that we have. I don't want to sound like a new age, therapeutic-touch self-help guru, putting everyone in touch with their inner child. But since we share a profession, I think I can help with the professional fears, the professional misperceptions. And these days, as we are constantly told about our inadequacies, I think it's a starting point.

So, my Christmas present to my fellow emergency physicians is my list of things you all do well, and ways in which you are excellent.

1) You are bright. Really bright. All of those years of college, medical school and residency weren't actually wastes of time. You are among the most capable and educated people in the history of medicine. You may sometimes feel like you aren't

intelligent. It isn't true. It only feels that way because you work in a setting where you must make far too many decisions in far too short a time. You are trying to understand your patients' afflictions in an isolated point in time without knowing them as a family doctor might. You are being forced to manage illnesses far too complex for the setting in which you work and far too difficult for the snapshot diagnosis and treatments expected of you today. You are expected to predict bad outcomes in people with seven complaints, ten existing medical conditions, eighteen medications and twenty-six allergies. It's a wonder they don't dissolve. Furthermore, the hopelessly complex patients who leave you full of doubt are frequently, and I mean this, lying. And if they aren't lying outright, they're so confabulated, so unwilling to assume responsibility, so helpless that they don't even know how to describe their problems. You, brothers and sisters, are brilliant. Because you work well in a situation that is very nearly impossible.

2) You are good. You care for people. You spend hours on a sexual assault exam, knowing that the case is hopeless because the victim doesn't actually know what happened, or who did it. She just knows she feels like she had sex. After she had sex with her boyfriend, that is. You try to help her. The police roll their eyes. You are good because you perform amazing professional contortions to find an alcohol rehabilitation center for a well known drunk who, once sober, gets angry because he didn't get jelly with his toast for breakfast, then leaves. You are good because you didn't try to find him and run over him with your SUV. You are good because you want so much to help the sick child, the beaten wife, the lost Alzheimer's patient, knowing full well that the situations are often lost causes. You are good because no one else in society would endure all of this knowing that they wouldn't be paid for the majority of it. Ask around. Hire the construction worker who owes you $5000 for fifteen "I need Lortab" visits. Contract him to remodel your house. When he finishes, tell him you

can't pay him. Hire a bodyguard. You, my friends, are so very good. Pity no one tells you very often.

3) You are brave. You walk into rooms where patients are violent from drug use, or are dripping their Hepatitis laden blood all over the floor and walls, screaming about the thug who stabbed them and who might yet come to visit. You try to calm and help them, never knowing which one will hit, stab or shoot you. You don't have the luxury of a bullet-proof vest or a sidearm. You recognize that your life may be taken as you try to help others who would pause only long enough steal your watch if they found you unconscious and bleeding out the eyes. You are willing to work during storms, riots, wars, terrorist attacks and epidemics. You are willing to work on St. Patrick's Day, Mardi Gras and New Year's Eve. That's brave. Outside of wartime, your courage finds few parallels.

4) You are gentle. You can leave the patient who just tried to punch you and touch the confused and frightened child with tenderness and sincerity. You can listen to the pain of someone who has just lost a loved one and in spite of your own weariness, actually care about them. Your hands have touched thousands of patients down their years and in each case you have tried to provide help or comfort. Few hands in the world can make that claim.

5) You are generous. Just look at how much you make on the dollar billed. You see everyone regardless of payment. You see them knowing that they owe you huge amounts of money. You see them knowing that they could sue you for millions having paid you nothing and that outside the profession, no one really cares. You do this willingly and even as you complain about EMTALA, you recognize that you are doing the right thing when so many physicians don't. If you knew how many patients you refer for outside care that don't get it (due to the $300 dollar up front charge) you would be aghast. Your generosity is impressive. And it isn't just the money. You sacrificed your youth to be physicians. You sacrifice your family to the schedule so that the department is always staffed.

You sacrifice your health to fatigue and your strength to the difficult challenges of caring for the sick and injured at all hours.

6) You are strong. Sure, you feel tired all of the time. The people you see make you tired. The schedule you keep is exhausting. Your body is not designed to be abused by the shifts you keep. Your mind is sharp, but so many decisions, so much information and so much sorting through half-truths leaves even the best brain weary. That you go back day after day makes you Herculean. Never look in the mirror and think you are weak. You couldn't do this if you were weak. This is a specialty where only the real women and men survive. Be proud. And do something restful for Heaven's sake.

7) You are not whiny, selfish or greedy. You ask and expect, very little compared with what you do. Society is glad to oblige your expectations.

8) You are not careless or dangerous. Your job simply places you in situations where people get sick and die. Considering the magnitude of your responsibilities, you should be expected to make mistakes. You seldom do.

So there it is. Merry Christmas! I'm proud of you all. Don't give up. Don't lie down in defeat. Don't let them abuse you or put you down, whether patient, administrator or fellow professional. You are too good to be treated badly. I'm sure there are lots of other good things I could say to you. But these are the ones I try to tell myself, I suppose. And don't think I've gone soft. I know none of us are perfect. In fact, I find myself becoming a little crazier every year. I'm proud of my neuroses. And I hope you are too, because you're all nuts. If you weren't, you'd be doing something else for a living.

Creatures of the Night

Here's to the creatures who roam the night
And sleep through the light of the day,
Here's to the creatures who drink and fight
And slur every word they say.

Here's to the beasties who need more drugs
For injuries no one can see;
Here's to the people with bites from bugs
And 'players' who burn when they pee.

Here's to the felons who never get tried,
For crimes that would make your blood cold;
Here's to the charm that cannot be denied
In the ladies who dance around poles.

Here's to the psychos, the dealers and slashers,
Who should be in cells without keys;
Here's to the rashes, the tattoos and gashes
That no one but us ever sees.

Here's to the madness, the sleepy eyed sadness
The restlessness, anger and lies;
Here's to the drama, the glory the madness,
The killer that blubbers and cries.

If I ever quit I am sure I would miss
All your stories and chaotic times;
'Cause hearing and seeing the things that you do
Gives meaning and life to my rhymes.

Ambiguity

A patient once complained to my group director that I had missed a fracture on X-ray. It was true. I had missed it. It was discovered by a radiologist who reviewed the films the next morning. The patient's comments were simply this "but it was broken!" No matter how my director tried to explain the subtleties of fractures and the ways in which they can be missed, this person only knew one reality. It was broken. Any fool could probably have seen that. In his mind there was a bone with a large crack across the middle separating it into two obvious pieces. There was apparently no ambiguity in the word 'broken.'

Unfortunately, there is ambiguity in medicine. Physicians don't like to admit it, although we do a better job now than we did many years ago. Patients don't like to believe it. They want certainty for their money. They want Marcus Welby or Dr. Green from ER. They want physicians to know the answers with unwavering confidence.

I wish I could always know the answer. It would make my shifts in the emergency department much happier. It would make me feel better when I discharge patients and when I leave work to go home. But it isn't going to happen. Because like it or not, human illnesses are not so easy.

I'm not a family practitioner. I don't have ongoing relationships with my patients (for the most part). So every person I see is a new puzzle. And some puzzles can be exhausting. Some stories seem so confusing that it almost feels as if some of my patients' illnesses or injuries happened to them without their knowledge and they suddenly materialized, sick or hurt, outside the door of the emergency department. When I introduce myself and ask "what's the problem tonight?" they answer "you're the doctor, why don't you tell me!" Sometimes they are too ill or simply don't have the words to put their symptoms into any coherent description. "It feels like I had this hot and cold water on my head and then my teeth all felt numb and everything around me looked small and shaky!" They didn't cover that in medical school.

This ambiguity is worse when compounded by alcohol. Doctors know that we have to be more careful with intoxicated persons. Their necks can be broken and they won't describe pain. They can have heart attacks and look restful. They can take other drugs and fail to tell us. And, like sober patients, they can simply elect to lie about their injuries or sicknesses, for fear that we will judge them, or for fear of legal difficulties.

All in all, medicine can be a very nebulous thing. The rock solid diagnoses we see on television are often hard to come by. Sometimes they are virtually impossible, as wave after wave of patients arrive with intoxication, suicide attempts, depression, heart failure, lung disease, broken faces, broken lives and hundreds of other maladies of body, mind and spirit.

So we keep looking because it's our job. We look for the big things, the obvious illnesses that can take patients to the grave. We look for the injuries hidden beneath bloody, mud caked clothes; for the chemicals hidden in the blood of unconscious patients; for the subtexts and agendas that accompany confusing, circuitous histories and which can reveal problems as severe as domestic violence or as trivial as the need for work excuses.

We sift through uncertainty in order to extend our patients' lives, to comfort them, to honor our profession and hopefully avoid errors that might be considered malpractice. But it can be difficult. Because what seems so clear the next day or in the court or in the newspaper may have been a thing that slipped under the radar of a harried provider in a busy practice; or that evaded someone caring for a patient with a complex disease, a confusing story or breath like a distillery.

The truth is the ambiguity of medicine is why we have that old saying about medicine being an art, not a science. Actually it's both. We need the internal, voiceless sense that the art brings as well as the knowledge and hope of the science. Only the combination keeps doctors on course in the face of so much illness, so much pain and so little clarity.

Aliens in Our Midst

I find myself caring for a great many aliens. They are legal and illegal, male and female, adult and child. They sometimes speak foreign languages, and their skin may not look like mine. Generally they are not identifiable by any superficial characteristic. I know they are aliens because as I treat them, I learn that they are citizens of difficult and troubled countries, whose borders lie all around my own safe and comfortable land. And I become immersed in their cultures every night in the emergency room.

I realized they were aliens when I read about them in the Bible. Exodus 22:21 says "Do not mistreat an alien or oppress him, for you were aliens in Egypt." Psalm 146:9 says "The Lord watches over the alien…" God himself watches over the dispossessed, sensitive as He is to wandering people in search of a better life. Scripture doesn't specify how they look or sound. I have found that the people I see, who live in fear and loneliness, are nothing more than aliens who come to the emergency room just to escape the wilderness of their lives.

Phil was one of them. Drunk on New Years Eve, he broke his hand in a fight. Cussing me for being too slow he paced the emergency room. When I finally sat down with him we had a little exchange, then came to an understanding. He was drunk he said, because he was going blind at age 23. Shoving his thumb deep into his already blind right eye he explained that the light would leave his left eye soon. His baby, two months old, was in the waiting room. He said he had to get drunk because it was all too much. A new baby and blind eyes unable to watch her grow up Phil lives full time in a land of enormous sorrow and drinks just to take away the edge. He came to me to have the pain taken away from his hand. But that was just the tip of the iceberg. He is an alien looking for a place where his body is whole and he is free of the terror of his blindness.

James was another. Sitting in camouflage pants and T-shirt, with messy brown hair and slouching posture, James was the typical rural Southern teen male. His South Carolina inflection made him no different from any of the young men I see in a shift. He came because of a rash. His grandmother told me the rest of his problems. "His momma's dead and his daddy's in prison." He was impassive. He knew the tragedy of his own story too well. He was an alien to the world where moms and dads raise children, where care and affection flow like rain on parched young men.

Sometimes my patients are hurled out of their worlds and into mine by sudden tragedy. I think of Roger, unable to move his legs after being shot in the spine by his lover's jealous boyfriend. "Will I walk again? Will I Doc?" I didn't know if he would. He had entered a world where violence was the price of passion. I don't know how many people from that world I have cared for, as men proved their manhood with fists and knives, as women were beaten for a sharp word, as children were shaken for crying. All of them aliens to safety. All of them looking for a place to sleep in peace.

I think of the many boys and girls I have seen whose lives are empty of the love they need. Ignored by parents for years they come to believe that they can only find security and tenderness by offering their bodies. Instead of playing games they play adult. Too soon, they are parents themselves without ever enjoying childhood or adolescence. The cycle continues as their infants are soon exiled from normal affection by the spiral of distrust, infidelity and rage that brought them into the world. I see these children and children's children, because of accidents, illnesses and sexually transmitted diseases. They are aliens using romance and passion as a rickety footbridge to the land of true love.

Danny was drunk every time I saw him. And every time, he wanted narcotics because his brother had "stolen" his prescription. He looked older than his 35 years, with tired eyes and lined face, his belly swollen with fluid as his liver died slowly of alcohol and drugs. The things he desired most were slowly killing him. I wonder how many days of his adult life he had been sober, with clear eyes and mind? He was an alien to clarity, to sobriety. He was a prisoner in a country of deadly things. He needed a land where he could be free of his addictions. Ultimately, he died a slave to the chemicals he wanted so much.

Russell threatened to kill all of us at one time or another. We expected to see him come in the back door with a shotgun some night. Thank God it never happened. Mostly he was just drunk. He would fight with the paramedics after he called them and clutch his chest for the 300th time, saying he was dying. He would scream profanities until we said, "Russell, there's a baby in the next room, please don't do that!" and he would cry and apologize. One of my partners heard him quote flawless sonnets by Shakespeare. Most of his adult life had been spent in prison. Russell even murdered a man there. What banished him from the land of the living? I never found out. Maybe his father was a drunk who beat him. Maybe he just met the wrong people. He was a tragic exile from the good things most of us enjoy, an alien to love, light, peace and health. I imagine that on the right path he would have been a doting father and grandfather, a teacher, a farmer, a mountain of a man who kept the nursery in church on Sunday morning. I know he loved his mother and friends. He cried out loud when we told him that his tattooed drinking buddy had died. Russell himself died of lung disease from smoking. We were aliens to one another I suppose. But I liked him and he liked me I guess. After all, he never actually killed me.

Amelia, at age 32, has diabetes so severe that she is blind. She is hospitalized every month or so and I sincerely doubt that she will ever reach 40. It's true that she never took care of herself when she was younger and newly diagnosed. She was frequently in the hospital with her glucose wildly out of control, then went home and ate candy like there was no tomorrow. She's pitiful now and it's partly her fault. But that doesn't mean she isn't one of God's children. She's simply an alien to health. She will never do the things that other women in their thirties do. She won't travel, exercise, or work. But God commands that like every alien, she be treated with kindness.

As a physician, I also forget how many of my patients are aliens to prosperity. I drive a nice car to the hospital; I live in a large house; I send my children to school each day in clean clothes without holes. But sometimes I get angry when patients return without having filled their prescriptions. But what can they do? Sometimes they could do better. They could stop smoking and drinking and use that money for their families. But many don't have a habit that robs them; they just have nothing. And I've seen a truckload of them in the rural South. They must feel like exiles, living as they do in a country so wealthy it sells gourmet dog food.

It isn't just the emergency room. Every day I pass aliens. Men and women and children whose lives are so far from mine that I could scarcely understand them. Their joys and sorrows unique and their troubles so terrible that my greatest problems seem trivial. They may be carrying guilt or pain, disease or sorrow. They may be lonely, depressed or mentally ill. They may be gay or straight, newborn or ancient, righteous or evil. God didn't make a distinction. He simply said to care for the aliens. It makes sense, really. Because if we follow Him, we remain aliens ourselves as long as we live on earth. All he wants us to do is look after our own. In the final analysis, everyone is the same. We are all traveling in search of the country that will finally be our home.

An Old Woman's Memories

I recall the little old lady lying on the hospital bed, sleeping quietly, her fretful, worried daughter sitting by the bed. Her daughter was concerned that her mother, well into her 90's, slept too much. That she was not herself and that she seemed to hallucinate. She told me her mother heard the voices of children and once told her that a little girl had slept all night in her bed. I later found an abnormality that suggested she might have cancer. What happened since, I have no idea. But I was intrigued by her hallucination, her delusion, or perhaps, her memory of sometime past.

You recall the story of the library at Alexandria. A vast repository of ancient knowledge, it was ultimately burned by the Romans in conquest and legend says the scrolls were used to heat Roman baths. This would seem to be a metaphor for each human life. Each life is an immense library of experience stored as memory. And it's useful to remember that each life that passes in the coming months is a collection of memories lost to our experience. It would be good to learn the unique value of each of those collections, more unique than snowflakes, more varied than the stars of the night sky and more precious than platinum.

We form these memories from the day of our birth; perhaps we form them in the womb or in some intangible place where we are spirit only, before our beginnings as cellular conglomerations. But every second of our lives that passes must somehow be placed, if only in a faint collection of signals and images, into our personal file, our personal mosaic and image of life. Imagine it. Every touch, every smell, every feeling, every slight, joy, hate, praise, pain or pleasure, put away for another time. If we could feel every one of those, if we could relive them, we would certainly go mad, for the sum of the experience would overwhelm our ability to assimilate. But in sequence, or in small doses, they are among our most treasured possessions. Coupled with our ability to imagine the future, our recollections of the past define us as human beings. And in that definition, create each life as an irreplaceable part of the tapestry of humanity as a whole.

I like to think that the lady I mentioned was living somehow in the past. That she recalled the childhood of her children and their laughter and that lying in her bed alone, she was warmed by the body of a child from long ago and whom she hoped to visit again soon. We view this as tragic in our society and somehow believe that the present, seasoned with hope for the future is the only possible existence. But memory is a heavenly grace. It blesses the healthy and the ill, the young and the old. I think that the elderly who see their end as surely as the sunset must find great solace in their dwelling place of antiquity. Everyone should have a hope for the future, but what of those who know the hope is frail? The terminally ill for instance. The past, so often viewed as water under the bridge, may well be the river to the sea of eternity, wherein all recollections are present and where memories become realities once more.

Someone once told me their belief that the feeling of deja'vu, that sense we have been somewhere before, is because time folds and turns upon itself and returns and returns like some artfully bowed ribbon. Others in my family believe that time is non-linear and that we in reality exist apart from it, the clock being only a poor tangible representation of our inability to perceive the infinity in which we dwell. I am not sure. But I believe that memory is more than some neurologic slide show that exists only to bore us to our death, like some relative's vacation photos. I think it is the repository of our being, taken apart and stored for us in small bits to remind us of the intense joys of life, of the sorrows that make us need hope. It exists so that it can one day be reconstituted in timelessness, allowing us not only to see it as images, but live it and feel it in its entirety and from each point to construct new and eternal images that defy our understanding of memory, time or reality. Maybe that is what Heaven is all about. I hope I get there and see the lady from the hospital bed reclining with a beautiful child, stroking her hair and telling her that they will never part again.

Compassion has a Price

A few nights ago, an elderly lady in our area began to have chest pain. Someone called 911. When the paramedics arrived at her home, she was stoic (as so many in her generation are) and was hesitant to come to the hospital. Ultimately she consented. When she arrived at Oconee Memorial, it became evident that she was having a heart attack. Unfortunately, it involved such a large area of her heart that she could not maintain an adequate blood pressure and was in shock.

We did as much as we could, as did our on-call cardiologist. She received a clot-dissolving thrombolytic drug. She received fluids and medication to support her blood pressure. She went to the cardiac catheterization lab, where she was found to have severe coronary artery disease. While there, our cardiologist attempted to place an intra-aortic balloon pump, a device which helps a sick heart to move adequate volumes of blood to the rest of the body. She continued to deteriorate, so she was transferred to the regional teaching hospital.

The next night, the nurses, medics and I learned that she had died. We were sad, of course, because we tried hard and because she and her family were gracious and good. We see a lot of patients whose complaints are relatively minor, so we become deeply involved when we have a fight on our hands. In spite of her death, we knew that everyone had done their best.

Looking back on this encounter, some might say that her care, given her age (over 70) and the severity of her disease, was too costly. In fact, it was costly. The thrombolytic drug alone costs a patient thousands of dollars. The cardiac catheterization costs thousands as well. The list goes on. We know that the majority of Medicare dollars are spent at the end of life and this was certainly true in her case. As a nation, we are faced with uncertainty about how to finance the future medical needs of a population that is growing, aging and has increasing expectations. Add to those concerns the yearly explosion of medical knowledge and the equation is hopelessly complex.

I'm no economist. I don't know what we should do about costs. Certainly there are patients, health care providers and institutions that abuse the system. But the overwhelming majority do not, so the fix doesn't lie in something as simple as stemming fraud. The government and private sector have been struggling for years to find a solution and neither seem to have the final answer. Maybe, as a nation, we're just crazy. All of that money could go to education or recreation. It could go to preventive health care, national defense or infrastructure. So why do we continue to pour money into acute health care?

Rather than ask ourselves what is wrong with the system we need to ask, for a change, what is right. And what is right is this: we still revere human life. We find ourselves, as a culture, unable to look our fellow human beings in the eye and say, "sorry, you don't get any more care; nice knowing you." It is a testament to our respect for the elderly and a reminder of our hope for the young. It speaks volumes about who we are.

As a nation we may be post modern, sophisticated and cosmopolitan, but we are still a people guided, deep in our collective heart of hearts, by a Judeo-Christian ethic that views life as divine in origin. And this ethic has thus far prevented us from dismissing life for purely financial reasons. One could argue that this practice has brought us too great a fiscal burden, but I don't think we would forgo it for that reason. Because compassion still defines us. And because we know that, for all the cost of medical care, we don't believe it is too expensive when we need it in the first person.

I'm sorry that my patient died. I'm sorry that her family is faced with loss and grief. But I'm thankful to her for reminding me that our struggle with sickness and death is worthwhile. And that our success cannot be measured against mortality which always wins. Our success, as a profession and a society should be measured by the triumph of compassion over callousness, humanity over utilitarianism. Because these victories are priceless.

Crazy is as Crazy Does

One of my very favorite movies is Jeremiah Johnson, starring Robert Redford. In one scene Johnson, a mountain man, has helped a woman to bury her dead family, killed by Indians. She is mad with grief and spends all of her time by their graves wailing. She doesn't speak, she only growls. Before going on his way, he says to her "Ma'am, the Indians will not bother you now, on account of you are touched". He means she is crazy and that her craziness will cause her attackers to view her with some respect and fear.

I think we have too long neglected the word crazy. Sadly, it has become a victim of modern political correctness, put away by the fashionable tendency of everyone to be offended by everything. It has been further displaced by the attempts of the medical profession to "medicalize" every aberrant behavior and life event. Still it is a word with immense utility in the field of emergency medicine. Because, dear brothers and sisters, we work with a population on the cutting edge of crazy.

Now don't get me wrong. I'm not actually referring to the mentally ill. I'm referring to those people who defy description. Men and women whose presentations render useless the DSM guidelines so revered by our psychiatric cousins. For instance, the lady who one night told me that all of her teeth had suddenly come loose, moved around and then locked back into place. If she was psychotic, she certainly didn't act that way. She was quite lucid and pleasant when I told her, as gently as I could, that what she described was impossible. I think she was just crazy.

Crazy also accurately describes some of the situations our patients find themselves in and from which we are expected to extricate them. Not long ago I saw a child who needed to be evaluated for sexual assault. Her assailant was an individual her parents had met at Wal-Mart. He claimed to be a cousin, visiting from Utah. They let him move into their home to "give him a chance", then after some two weeks allowed him stay with their toddler daughter while they were out of the house. A neighbor, apparently stopping by at 2:00 a.m. for heaven knows what, allegedly saw the child being molested. When the family came home the fur flew, as the neighbor, husband and child's mother all attacked the alleged assailant. The ambulance brought three patients. Cousin Utah, with two broken forearms; mom with a boxer's fracture of the hand and a child in need of a sexual assault exam. Crazy is as crazy does.

As if I need to drive the point home, there was the man whose chief complaint involved something like a dream sequence in the shower, which was co-hosted by Homer Simpson. He said to the nurses, "it wasn't erotic, or anything". What a relief. That would have turned crazy into frankly disturbing.

I also believe that crazy is a useful term for those patients who bear diagnoses that are popular, but nebulous at best. I don't need to name the diagnoses. We all know what they are. Unfortunately they are a growing portion of my practice. Invariably, they end up under the care of a physician who is also crazy (and often unavailable for consultation). They come to emergency departments in an attempt to pull me into their delusion by asking for bizarre and unsubstantiated treatments recommended by their doctor. Maybe they have real illnesses, but most of the time there are neither objective findings of nor scientific explanations for their problems. I think this is because physicians fail to confront them with what would probably be a liberating truth: "Sir, in my professional opinion, you're just crazy!"

This sounds harsh, but isn't. I mean, in times past crazy people were well-respected members of any village or community. People deferred to them. They helped them financially. They humored them and left them alone. They were often felt to be a little closer to the divine than your average person, which made their behavior seem more respected and more tolerable. It was as if their experience of the ineffable made them understandably off-center. Crazy wasn't always such an insulting proposition.

Of course, I don't know how we would code it. It isn't in the index of major medical texts. It doesn't have diagnostic criteria like schizophrenia, bipolar disorder, stroke or pelvic fracture. It isn't visible on x-ray, and evades even the most comprehensive laboratory panels. The diagnosis of crazy is one that requires some subjective use of personal experience. It can be exceptionally hard to apply during medical school and residency, when one's personal library of patient encounters is relatively limited and when premature application of the diagnosis can result in embarrassing experiences on morning rounds, as real pathology parades as craziness. But after a few years in practice it becomes clear that the diagnostic criteria are both indescribable and plain as day.

I have a friend who says that on the last day of his practice, when he retires to blissful, constant fishing, he will go from room to room and tell everyone exactly what he thinks about them and their problem. A good man, I'm sure he will reserve his ire for those who have truly earned it. But I suspect that one of the things he will say as he moves happily from patient to patient will be "crazy, that's what you are. Always have been, always will be." I hope I'm there to see it. Even better, maybe I'll be crazy by then too.

Barbarians are Alive and Well

On a recent emergency department shift I saw a young man who had been to a sorority formal with his girlfriend. On the way home, another couple entered the bus that they were riding on campus. The second woman, in her formal dress, was forced by her date to sit on the floor of the bus while he sat in what was apparently the last seat. My patient offered up his seat to the damsel on the floor. Her date attacked him, fracturing the bones of his face and knocking him unconscious.

It was refreshing to be reminded that chivalry lives. But it was disconcerting to be reminded, once again, that barbarism is alive and well. The word barbarian has its roots in ancient Greek civilization. It originally referred to someone who could not speak Greek and was thus uncivilized. It has since been used to refer to those who were uncultured or unlearned; sometimes it is used as an insult to refer to groups or individuals felt to be inferior. It's origins were further defined for me when I once read a reference by an etymologist who believed that it was originally a form of verbal mockery, with the sound "barbar" being somehow an imitation of a foreign and confusing tongue. Word origins are useful in this case because I believe that the word barbarian fits the aforementioned attacker quite nicely.

First, to use the term in its most insulting form, such behavior is indicative of an inferior character. Is this a value judgment? Absolutely. I make it with neither hesitation nor guilt. As a nation we have been too long indoctrinated into the belief that every person's behavior is ultimately excusable for any one of a number of reasons: they were raised poorly, they were unhappy, they were intoxicated, addicted, spurned, shunned or spoiled. While I recognize that persons often behave poorly for complex reasons and sometimes need help to overcome the causes of such behavior, it would be a mistake for us to view felonious activity as tolerable in the name of kindness and understanding. To do so would negate the entire criminal code.

Second, the word barbarian describes the person in question because this language of violence is foreign; its vowels and consonants are hard on the ear. They sound like gibberish. It is a language spoken by persons unlearned in the ways of right behavior, uncultured in the ways

30

of civilized society. Barbarism has little to do with level of education or income. I have seen it in educated persons with good jobs, as well as those who were poor and illiterate. Barbarism cannot be characterized by simple descriptors of dollars and degrees, regions or heritage.

Later that same evening, my patient's assailant was brought in by police. He was laughing, exhibiting no concern for what he had done. But someone that night was concerned. The man in handcuffs had a gash in his head, caused by others on the bus who pulled him off of his chivalrous victim. In short, he was attacked by those who viewed his behavior as beneath contempt. While I oppose vigilantism and detest mobs, I can only say "Bravo!" Bravo to those with the courage to act in defense of the innocent. Bravo to the young man who showed his fellow students the meaning of another word, gallantry.

Later, I received a subpoena to testify as a witness for the prosecution in an assault case from last year. I had seen the victim as a patient. Although I was initially annoyed, grumbling to myself about going to court on my day off, it occurred to me that this was the necessary price of punishing the very behaviors I find most disturbing, having spent far too many hours tending to the results of violence. I realized that it was not only my civic duty to appear at the courthouse that day, it was an honor to be included in a case which might just make the world a little bit safer, if only for a while, from one more barbarian.

Even Doctors Get Sick

We should all be sick. Every doctor occasionally, just as a reminder of who and what we are. I have been lately. I can say that it's more than an insight into our patients' lives. It accomplishes more than some sensitive epiphany about caring and profession. Sickness is somehow sublime.

This year I have tried on several sicknesses. I don't think I'm a hypochondriac, because they've been objectively discernable problems. And I don't think I really want to be invalid or disabled, because I dislike inactivity. But I have enjoyed, on some odd level, each experience.

In January came the ankle sprain. While teaching Tae Kwon Do class I kicked, stepped down and rolled my ankle. There was a sound. Was it a pop? A snap? A tear? I didn't know. But I knew I couldn't stand on it. Like every good physician, I did nothing except limp and complain. No x-rays, no splint, no crutches. I was going to take my wife and children skiing in West Virginia and not even a fractured ankle would stop me. But now and then, the tenderness and growing purple discoloration of my foot made me wonder if my technique of therapeutic denial wasn't, maybe, short sighted. In the end, I was better. It only took about eight weeks.

But my body wasn't finished with insights. Not long after came the kidney stone. It was my second. By the second, the pain is clearly recognizable. Sitting having breakfast with my daughter, the devil himself took my kidney in hand and squeezed it, like someone making kidney juice for breakfast in hell. At our hospital, I slipped quietly, calmly, into the relief that morphine brings. The next day, when the pain ambushed me during work, I slipped happily into the sweet, dreamless peace of Demerol. Ah, Demerol. And pher-pher-phan, or whatever I called Phenergan that night as I staggered to the car and said goodbye to chuckling nurses. My kidney stone reminds me of just how bizarre pain can be. Pain, so universal, so overwhelming is a thing that unites every human in a way just short of the commonality of our deaths. How almost delightful when we feel it! How even more delicious its absence. Oddly, I can't even remember which side it was on.

But when it comes to really appreciating illness, there's nothing like a good pneumonia. I'm writing this in Denver, about to go on a retreat, getting over a pneumonia that began in South Carolina as what I assumed was a pollen allergy and culminating in the emergency department at Mayo Clinic Hospital, Scottsdale, Arizona. It has been quite a little odyssey.

I was in Scottsdale to speak, but with each day there I struggled more and more to breathe. When I finally admitted that I was sick, finally accepted that those had been chills, finally faced the possibility I could be ill, I found that I had a fever of 101 and pneumonia in my left lung, exactly where I felt it. Antibiotics, steroids and inhalers later, I'm better. But now, having flown from Arizona to this rather lonely hotel in Denver, I find that my improvement didn't quite account for altitude. I feel a new understanding of the purse-lipped old men and women who ride into the emergency room on gurneys, or who roll back in wheelchairs. It's a terrifying irony, an awful corporal betrayal, that one can be immersed in oxygen rich air but unable to use it. It's to be a starving man with no mouth, seated at a banquet.

So I have experienced a lot so far this year. I have felt narcotics race through my brain to help me ignore my screaming flank. I have wondered if I'd ever have a normal ankle again. I have lain awake at night in a hotel far from home, with a kind of manic insomnia (from inhalers and steroids) that made my hands too tremulous even to type on my computer for the comfort that writing brings. I approach my 40th birthday facing my frailty as a human creature, my fear of disability, my susceptibility to loneliness.

But I also face my humanity. I face my strength. I face the blessings of health care, the rich rewards of living in a society where science exists to make us live longer than we should. In my little journey this year, this week, I face my patients. Sickness teaches doctors as much as any lecture or text ever did. Sickness teaches us what it feels like to need a doctor, what it feels like to wonder, to be uncertain, to be actually afraid. Sickness makes us understanding. And however bad it feels, it always has a lesson if we pay attention.

Still, I said at the beginning that sickness isn't just a festival of wisdom and empathy. Sickness is like everything else that faces us. An experience that is inevitable. And sometimes it's important just to embrace it, however briefly, before we go on with our lives.

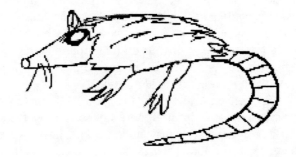

The Big Possums Walk the Night

Spring and summer weekends always seem to be the same in the Oconee Memorial Hospital Emergency Department. The EMS radio chatters the same codes over and over. Signal 13, signal 45, code 6. (Laceration, intoxicated, altercation). I typically drive in on Friday and Saturday nights to see a parking lot full of young people smoking and laughing while friends are seen as patients. I guess if you hang out in the hospital parking lot, eventually you're bound to see something interesting.

One recent shift I was bemoaning the fact that so many bad things happen at night. I was talking about this to my good friend, Sgt. Neal Brown of the SC Highway Patrol. He summed up the problem. "You see Ed, the big possums walk at night," he said succinctly. Andy Griffith couldn't have said it better.

As such, I would like to briefly call on my interesting, but generally unused, zoology degree to explain why it's wise to avoid the big opossums at night. You see, opossums are among the oldest and most successful of all mammals in the world. They have successfully reproduced and lived in almost every environment on earth. They are mostly nocturnal. They will eat virtually anything. Except for their strange propensity to walk out in front of moving vehicles, they seem to have amazing survival instincts. But they can be mean. Ask anyone who's ever accidentally encountered one in the dark, seen it's gleaming eyes and sharp teeth in the flashlight, then heard it hiss in anger. Little wonder that some mornings the dog is limping on a bloody leg and the cat, atop the woodpile, looks stunned from the opossums well meaning, but misguided, amorous intentions.

So how can we apply this to human behavior? There are some big opossums out there, my friends. I hope to instill this understanding in my boys as they grow into adventurous manhood, as well as in any reader who tries to learn by reflection instead of experience. The big opossums like to fight. They'll fight anyone, anytime, for something as slight as an annoyed look. They don't have the same sharp teeth, (although they do bite), but rest assured they have no compunction about slashing, stabbing, beating or shooting anyone who gets in their way. They have a gleam in their eye that is usually brighter when intoxicated. They are resilient. They'll roll their car over a mountain, break multiple extremities and walk out of the hospital against medical advice. They seem to undergo almost weekly violent injuries and go back to the same watering hole for more of the same. I have said and still maintain, there are some people you just can't kill. Mutual of Omaha's 'Wild Kingdom' could have devoted months to this species. "Watch as Jim attempts to come between the giant two legged opossum and his potential mate! Notice as Jim tries to avoid the broken beer bottle!"

They are a truly fascinating species. To their credit, I haven't found many that I couldn't get along with and I see a lot of them. All I try to do is show them respect, maintain a reasonable distance and make it evident that I am not a threat. (Of course, other standard rules apply, like don't move suddenly, don't surprise them and don't leave food, money or prescription drugs lying around).

The big opossums are a part of the social milieu of America that will never go away. Although potentially dangerous, many of them are hard working individuals who just let go a little on weekends. Any other time they're as nice as pie. They often do the jobs no one else wants, but that we all recognize as necessary. As such, I suppose they deserve a little fun. I just wish it didn't always involve drinking and fighting.

The bottom line is this. The world is dangerous enough; we all know that. So it makes sense to avoid those situations and groups which increase our personal risk. My mom and dad used to say that there wasn't anything worthwhile going on after midnight. Now I see how right they were. Because after midnight, the big opossums walk the earth. And they are a species to reckon with.

A Little Summer Fun

Every spring I look for the patient whose actions will set the tone for the vacation season to come. It's kind of a game because even as I view the coming months with some horror, I am continually entertained by the parade of injuries and illnesses that the hot days and nights bring.

I think I have a winner. Recently, as I listened to the EMS dispatcher, I heard a report that assured me it would not be a dull season. Two patients were coming to the emergency department who had been involved in a riding lawnmower accident. It was 11pm. This caught my attention. Fortunately neither seemed severely injured as they rolled through the door. The woman involved had simply been trying to help her injured husband. Her husband, the driver of the vehicle, possessed the chagrined look of a man who knew that what he did was a little, well, out of the ordinary.

When I quizzed him about the accident all he would do was smile and say, "I'd rather not talk about it." Eventually he told me that he had just bought a brand new riding mower and even though it was pitch black outside, he just had to take it for a spin. During that little spin he rolled it. Fortunately he did well, although he sustained more significant injuries than were initially apparent. His wife, minimally injured, will no doubt have "I told you so" deeply ingrained in his mind for years to come.

What is it about spring and summer? Why do we do the things we do? As I look back on my career to date I can safely say that humans behave with an alarming predictability this time of year. We eat too much, drink too little (water, that is), seldom wear sun-screen and regularly test the patience of stinging insects and biting reptiles. We consistently forget that our bare feet are no match for nails or glass shards. And as a species, we become more than ever susceptible to the ancient belief that the mixture of alcohol and sunshine produces a kind of mystical force field protecting us from any and all injuries, whether induced by automobiles, chainsaws, knives or bullets.

Motorized vehicles, land based or aquatic, seem to have an allure that is almost chemical during the summer months. Men especially seem genetically linked to combustion engines, seeking every possible means to attach their bodies to them for the purpose of high-speed propulsion. Admittedly this can be great fun; however it seems more than ever an integral part of natural selection as the earth tilts into the sun's intensity. I myself have been counseled by my dear, wise wife to pay more attention and try not to cross the bow of large craft so closely while riding a jet-ski. (In clear illustration of my point, I did not even realize the large craft was present at the time. My XY chromosome combination was obviously trying to remove me from the gene pool).

Another phenomenon observed by anyone in medicine or law enforcement is the clear increase in violence in spring and summer. I have a theory that holds that humans, like molecules, simply bump into each other more as the temperature rises and that dangerous reactions occur as they meet with increasing frequency. Although some reputable social scientists might consider my view simplistic, I stand firm. I have definitely seen more stabbings, shootings and beatings in the hotter months. When we combine heat, excess alcohol, drugs, and boredom, then stir evenly, we have an explosive concoction that makes diesel fuel and fertilizer look like a box of cherry bombs.

Nevertheless, I'm ready to run the gauntlet. The onslaught of maddening behaviors is completely unavoidable. Spring is winding down and summer looms large and scary before me. Like St. George, I need to ride like mad at the dragons of soaring mercury and falling IQ points. So fetch me the shirtless and shoeless! Bring on the heat-stricken masses smelling faintly of barbecue sauce and tequila! I am unafraid. I am capable. And I am really looking forward to autumn.

The Voices in My Head

I'd like to say that I'm always focused on patient care. I'd like to say that every word that patients say to me in the emergency department is taken seriously and given weight. But I'd be lying. Because inevitably, when the story goes on and on, when the complaint becomes lost in meaningless information, my mind just wanders away. I suspect we all do it from time to time. We drift off to distant places or bizarre thoughts (some more distant and bizarre than others). So here's a little transcript of a patient interaction, taken from inside my head, just to illustrate my point:

Background: Mr. Peterson is an articulate, fastidious man of 46 years. His chief complaint is, initially, abdominal pain. He is sitting quietly on the side of the examining table, his black socks pulled tightly up to his knees, hands clasped on his lap. His hair is combed and his teeth are brushed. He doesn't have a single prison tattoo visible. His stylish but understated wife, in pink sweat suit and matching running shoes, sits in the corner reading a historical romance novel. As I walk into the exam room I think, "Score! A normal, non-mutant human being with a medical problem that I can solve! Let the healing begin!"

Au Contraire

Mr. Peterson: Hello doctor. I'm very glad to see you. We've been waiting 28 minutes and 3 seconds. But that's neither here nor there. I've been having pain for a long time. According to my records it's 8 months and 4 days. What I get is this tingling, burning feeling in my stomach that goes down to my groin and around my back. Sometimes it actually takes my breath.

What I say: Does anything make it start? Eating particular foods, or activity? Does it radiate into your testicle?

What I think: Hmm, maybe an ulcer? Maybe he has biliary colic? Kidney stones are a possibility. I'll have to check a urine.

Mr. Peterson: Funny you should ask. It always gets worse at exactly 2:15 in the afternoon, then again at 3:00 in the morning, on the dot. Here, I'll show you. I keep a log with the time it started, how long it lasted, what I was doing during the attack and the local weather conditions.

What I say: Thanks! That could be helpful. I'll look it over. Is there anything you're doing at those times? Straining, lifting? Also, are you an engineer by any chance?

What I think: Uh-oh

Mr. Peterson: Not really. I mean, at 2:15pm I have my afternoon protein bar while I take 13 minutes for a work break, but in the early morning, I'm either asleep or on the Internet. Another thing you might want to know: When I get the pain I cough three times. Exactly. And sometimes my left eye gets a little blurry. And yes, I am an electrical engineer. Why do you ask?

What I say: It doesn't really sound food related. Do you get anxious or upset at those times? That could contribute to stomach upset. Do you get short of breath when you cough? Does your headache give you blurred vision?

What I think: Sounding less serious. Too many complaints to unify into one dangerous entity. Hang on man, focus. Don't let go of the moment, be a doctor!

Mr. Peterson: I'm not crazy. No, I've been reading on several websites and this isn't anxiety related. However it may correspond to a cyclic rupture of a parasite, like malaria. I'd like to be checked for that, if you would. I haven't left the country, but Malaria was once endemic to this area. And with bio-terrorism, well, you know anything could happen! (His wife looks up as if pleading for a swift death, rolls her eyes and returns to the well-muscled, swarthy, Seamus and the rocky slopes of Ireland.) I get a little short of breath, but it's very brief; about five seconds. I get a headache and yesterday I'd have to say it was the worst headache of my life, like a thunderclap almost. Yes, in fact I think I passed out.

What I say: Malaria, huh? (Then, quietly, Did you consider schistosomiasis?) Let's talk about your headache. You say it was the worst of your life?

What I think: Too late. Help, slipping... Boy, I wonder what the weather is like in Alaska right now. I need to go back and hunt again next year. The snow is probably falling already. Snow...I should also start looking for a place to take the kids tubing this winter. Is that engineer guy still talking? Of course he is. I'll bet his wife takes Xanax like candy.

Mr. Peterson: (human sounds, voice-like, then becoming clearer as my brain identifies that someone is speaking)...of course...beat up in grade school...and you bet it was. As a matter of fact, I have a log-book that records my headaches since 1989. I have every one logged, along with my evaluation and treatment. Do you think I need a lumbar puncture? I'd be very curious to know what my opening pressure is and how it compares to my last one. Have you ever heard of pseudo-tumor?

What I say: A log-book? Fascinating! May I see it? By the way, you don't exactly fit the profile for pseudo-tumor. Are there migraines in your family?

What I think: I have a headache now. Why, if I had a hammer I'd club myself. If I had a hammer, I'd hammer in the morning, I'd hammer in the evening, all over this land... Maybe his wife is trying to kill him slowly. There she is, in the corner trying to disappear. I wish I were reading a book, too. I'll try and communicate with her telepathically... Hey, Janet has a new scrub top! That's a nice color on her. It's very feminine. She's funny. I loved it when she told that guy he should floss his tooth! Boy, I wonder what we should get to eat tonight? Chinese might be good. I really need a Coke. If I were in France could I drink wine on the job?

Mr. Peterson. .... migraines... know I'm not classic, but according to...I could... because..... when.... child.... ferret.... meningitis.... my personal research on the Internet... wife said.... orchids... should... but, you know all about that I'm sure... Viagra... What do you think?

What I say: What?
What I think: What?

Mr. Peterson: I said, do you think I might have lymphoma? (Wife slips down in chair, feigning unconsciousness).
What I say: Well, I don't think so. Have you had weight loss or night sweats? I mean, let's CT your abdomen and look, so we'll both feel better. Your headaches sound rather chronic. I think, personally, that Malaria is an outside shot, considering you've spent your entire life in Clemson, South Carolina. But hey, I could be wrong. So let's do a smear and look for it.
What I think: Good save! Doesn't anyone recognize irony or sarcasm anymore? I know, we could put an X-Box in the lounge? Ghost Recon would be cool on night shift. I'm hungry. Good grief, I've only been here an hour. What is this, some kind of twisted time warp, where I just keep looping back on myself? Am I stuck forever with this man's personal medical charts? That would have been a good Twilight Zone. Maybe it could be a sci-fi novel? I think I'll go start writing it while I wait on the labs and CT.

Mr. Peterson: Are you going to examine me?
What I say: Absolutely. Let's try and make you feel better.
What I think: As if...hey, is that chocolate on the desk? Why is it that there's never a code-blue or cardiac arrest when you need one?

Mr. Peterson: Your hands are cold. How long have you been a doctor? Where did you go to medical school? Do you have a copy of your license I can see? I'd like you to show me all of my x-rays. My entire body is numb, did I tell you that?
What I say: I'm going to listen to your heart so don't talk for an hour. I mean a few seconds.
What I think: This guy is pale. Really pale. A little sunshine might help there, Casper. Casper. I love cartoons. Especially Foghorn Leghorn! Where am I again? Oh no, wherever it is, he's still here!

Making Sense of Loss

Driving out of the hospital last week, I turned onto the highway toward my house and family. I noticed the broken glass that littered the road in front of me. It was fine glass, almost a powder like the glitter that little girls love to play with. It was glass from a car wreck that claimed the life of a little girl, age five, who had been a K-4 classmate of my son, Samuel. I was not working the day she came to the hospital and I'm glad. I have had difficulty dealing with the emotions of that tragedy and I wasn't even there.

As I drove toward home, I passed Oconee Christian Academy, where she was to begin first grade this year, just like Samuel. I'm not sure what I thought. But I thought of her and of her absence and of the void in the world because she was not here anymore. And I drove home to my children. But she has been on my mind and so has her mother. Because I just don't understand it all.

I think about her and I think about the people I see in my practice in the emergency room. I think about the drunk drivers who take their own lives for granted, as well as the lives of others. I think of how they roll their vehicles over, are thrown from them and walk away with negligible injuries.

I recall the spouse abusers who beat senseless persons they vowed to love. I realize that they often live long lives, untroubled by any of the suffering they visit on others.

I consider the blissfully ignorant who would rather be dragged behind an angry bull than hold a job and how they drain society of resources it cannot afford to lose, all the while wasting day after day, at best watching television and getting more obese by the minute.

I see, in my memory's eye, the drug abusers who lie to me in ways I would never even have imagined, who break their bones intentionally to receive another prescription for narcotics and to whom the idea of quitting is simply out of the question.

And I think about persons who have heart disease and after life saving surgery continue to smoke one to two packs of cigarettes per day, spitting in the face of the gift of life they received.

This little girl was sitting in a car, full of potential, full of years of life and love and her reward was untimely death. I wonder why. Is it because God gives extra years to the evil and the ignorant, so that they have time to reconcile to him and use their lives well? Most likely, it is for a complex web of reasons I couldn't fathom even if I knew them. The thing is, I could use this sort of madness as a reason not to believe in God. It wouldn't be hard. Men and women have done it for ages. Suffering, they reason, means God cannot exist.

Frankly, it makes sense on a certain level. But my problem is, I have to believe because if I don't, the universe is a cruel amalgam of senseless horror, love, memory and desire. Sometimes I don't want to believe. But I have no alternative. If I don't believe, there isn't any hope that the little girl and her mother endured pain for any reason. And there isn't any hope they'll ever be together again. And if I don't believe, then whatever pain I will feel in the future is worthless and exists only because it does. It will have no purpose. And I will simply be a creature evolved with the non-adaptive ability to feel agony, combined with the illusory sense that somehow, tragedy shouldn't exist. It doesn't make sense. If tragedy weren't an abnormal state, then death would seem little more than a leaf fallen from a tree, rather than the universe rending thing it is.

I believe because I don't know how else to cope. But I want some answers someday. If I make it to heaven's gates, after railing against God like this (and I'm sure I will again), I'll be happy. But I'll also want to talk to the big guy. All of those "why's" will hopefully have reasons more satisfactory than "because". I believe God is rational. I look forward to the day when he shows me how much.

Oh to be Obsolete

I hope to be obsolete someday. This is an odd statement coming from a physician, I realize. But I write this sitting in the library at the University of Arizona Medical Center in Tucson. I am in town to give some lectures at a continuing education course. And it's good for me to be reminded of what a research center looks like, to rediscover the fact that my profession is supported and advanced by the efforts of researchers around the world. It is uplifting and a little disturbing to recognize that medicine is constantly moving forward and that even the best effort at continuing education leaves a physician practicing with knowledge several years behind the times.

As emergency physicians, my colleagues and I practice a type of medicine that makes us "jack of all trades, master of none". We operate in a limited window of time and make decisions based on a limited amount of information available on each patient. I believe we give excellent care.

But sometimes, as I step back and look at what we do, I am stricken dumb by the sheer inadequacy of modern medicine as a whole. Like all sciences, medicine must be constantly advanced, the void of ignorance filled with new knowledge. Like all arts, it must sometimes take off in completely unexpected directions. There is no holding steady. All pauses in learning are losses. Although I am not a researcher (nor does my personality leave me much risk of becoming one) I can recognize the immense value of research and scientific pursuit. I see its value in the needs of my patients to overcome complex and life-altering illnesses. I see its value in the eyes of my family as I worry what I will do if illness befalls them. And every year as I age and feel another pain, I know that the time will come when I too will hope for some breakthrough, perhaps for Parkinson's Disease which made my grandfather shake and may lie in wait for me.

So often we are at a loss in patient care. How does one treat pain in the cancer patient, yet allow them the clarity to enjoy their loved ones? How does one tell a mill worker that his hand cannot be reattached and it will never touch his child again? What do we say to reassure the

45

stroke victim, whose treatment with "clot busting" thrombolytic drugs may prove fatal?

We in medicine are not ignorant; we are only blindfolded by time. I hope for a day when medicine will have made great strides; great enough that needles and scalpels are the stuff of museums. A day when cancer is diagnosed and eradicated on the same office visit and when pain no longer holds its place in our psychic pantheon of fear, second only to death. I hope that if my children enter medicine as a profession, I will be virtually unable to understand the knowledge, techniques, devices and drugs at their disposal, so that I will shake my gray head and think with nostalgia about how it was in "the good old days".

I have an image in my mind of hospitals and clinics, empty and of my steps echoing as I tour down long, empty white halls that smell of years of antiseptic, an aged veteran of a long forgotten war. Of walking past empty ICU's, where patients no longer hold to the faint thread of life cast by imperfect medicine. Of opening the door of a chapel that no longer rings with the sobs of families, suddenly empty from the loss of a loved one to unstoppable illness or injury.

I believe that day will come; I also believe the ultimate fulfillment of my vision will have more to do with the Kingdom of God on earth that with the skill of science. But one can hope. Medicine must persevere and struggle, so that a thousand years hence, our professional descendants will look back on our practice with a shudder and a chill and whisper in hallowed classrooms the word "barbarians". Then we will have done the right thing as a science, as an art and as lovers of humankind.

Rural Practice

I practice in a place of expansive lakes, white-water rivers and the mist covered foothills of the Blue Ridge Mountains. The area includes thousands of acres of Sumter National Forest. The natural beauty is breathtaking. Sumter National Forest and our various state and county parks are laced with hiking trails; which are full of unique plants and trees, some found nowhere else. Fish and game abound. In fact, our wooded hospital grounds support a flock of at least 30 wild turkey. And last deer season, the only deer I saw were the three does grazing at the end of the ED driveway one night, spotlighted by two of our paramedics.

We have a lot of wonderful things here, things that are gifts of the rural life. We have good people, the salt of the earth types who care about personal morality and Southern courtesy. People who bring you a glass of sweet tea when your car breaks down. We live with a low crime rate and less illicit drug use than more populated areas. It is a good place to raise children. It's also a cool place to practice, where a busy summer shift can bring an acute MI, a near drowning (from inner-tubing on Class IV white water while drunk), a pit viper bite, a bull goring and many other pathologies, more or less interesting.

But as physicians in a rural area, we pay a price. Because we have to endure a certain stigma that says if you practice in a small, rural hospital, you must be less than competent. Because if you were competent; you'd practice in a large, urban teaching/trauma center. I frequently face this when I speak to the out of state parents of local university students. You can tell that they are hesitant. Many are from the urban northeast and they exude a discomfort with any physician willing to put out a shingle in a place so far off the beaten path. They want to know about the hospital, the consultants, my training, etc., Of course, this is fine. I understand that anyone might want to know the credentials of the person caring for their sick or injured child. But, as emergency physicians, I think we should try to dispel this unfortunate stereotype among patients. And the best place to start is to dispel it among our colleagues.

I read some time ago of the difficulty rural areas have in recruiting residency trained emergency physicians. I'm not surprised. Our training, mostly in large urban centers, tends to focus us on that type of medicine. We see trauma care as effective only when provided by trauma teams. We feel that cardiac care must be supported by immediate angioplasty and if needed, cardiac surgery capabilities. We love to hear the thump-thump of those helicopter blades. Our hearts thrill at the thought of thoracotomies (opening the chest with a scalpel and rib-spreaders for the non-medical) for gunshots and stabbings. We sometimes even buy the line that children have to be cared for in children's hospitals. We like to see herds of residents and students descend to the department to evaluate admissions in the early morning hours. It's shiny and exciting and it's very hard to resist.

I must admit I was a victim of the myth myself at first. When I first came to Oconee Memorial Hospital seven years ago, I was happy about the job. But somewhere, deep inside I felt that I had taken the low road. I felt that if I were "a real doctor", I'd have gone to a trauma center in a large city. And no wonder I moved to a town of 5000 persons. I became the fifth doctor in our group, seeing some 27,000 patients per year in a 10 bed ED, in a 120 bed hospital. We had one cardiologist but no cath lab. We had no neurologist, pulmonologist, neurosurgeon, toxicologist, trauma team or pediatric subspecialties. We had nine ICU (intensive care unit) beds and four telemetry beds. Although our group, our department and our hospital staff have grown dramatically since the time I arrived, it was and still is a far cry from Methodist Hospital of Indiana where I trained. Thankfully, my residency training prepared me well for the adventure of rural emergency medicine.

Here's why. In my rural department, in this relatively isolated area, my partners and I have to practice a very autonomous form of emergency medicine. We don't have residents to help with the volume and we don't have a trauma team. Until recently there was no helicopter service taking our patients to the regional trauma referral center; it's at least 40 minutes away by ground. We still lack many of the support specialties I listed above. Most nights we are the **only** physicians in the hospital. We have to manage the difficult airway, obtain the emergent vascular access, make the transfer arrangements and all the rest. Like physicians at many rural centers, we do it all. Of course, this is not really different from many emergency physicians in urban areas, but the difference is, we don't have options. We are relatively alone.

But my point is not to pat my own back. My point is that all across the country, physicians at small hospitals provide excellent, state of the art care for patients that are just as sick as the ones in large centers. But they do so with less help, less resources and in many ways more pressure than their friends and classmates in teaching centers. The view from the large centers sometimes gets skewed because only the sickest patients are transferred to them. So it sometimes looks like the smaller facilities do a bad job. Actually, most of them give great care. But patients deteriorate and patients die in hospitals of every size. It happens at Oconee Memorial and it happens at Methodist.

Our specialty should encourage graduating residents to go to rural areas. I'd like to see residents taught that they can contribute to the specialty as certainly in a remote area as they would in any large city in America. There is enormous need and there are great rewards in making a rural area safer and healthier. There is tremendous satisfaction in being appreciated by patients who might have done poorly if not for modern emergency care. When my family and I drive home to West Virginia, through rural Appalachia, I often wonder who is staffing the departments nearby, should we become intimate with a coal truck. I always hope it's someone well trained for the job.

Rural areas require that physicians sacrifice certain big city amenities, both professionally and socially. But the payoff is worth it. And if anyone reading this is considering rural emergency medicine, I encourage them to make a difference and go to the country. They won't regret it; I certainly don't.

The Blessed Mundane

Both my grandma Leap and my grandpa Owens had a peculiar tendency that began after they became bound to nursing homes as a result of strokes. They cried. They cried readily, without any obvious reasons, usually when family would visit, then prepare to leave. They would stumble through conversations, straining to hear our words as their stricken brains failed to support their tongues, failed to process the sounds their ears brought to them. They would laugh some and hold our hands. They would sit quietly and look at us with deep love. They would attempt to hug us when we came close. But always, at some point, they began to weep.

They were not sad persons before that time. Grandma Leap was a woman of vigor, raised on a farm in Lincoln County, West Virginia. She endured the depression, faced the loss of siblings, parents and husband and raised three fine sons. She worked daily in her home, yard and garden. She was widely read, deeply devout and exceptionally fun.

Grandpa Owens was the son of a teamster who built roads in West Virginia using horse drawn equipment. Grandpa loved and kept horses all his life. He cared deeply for his wife and daughter. He worked hard as a truck driver until his retirement and had friends and family all across West Virginia, Kentucky and Ohio.

But something happened when my grandparents began their medical incarceration. I could imagine any number of reasons for their tears. Perhaps they were tears of loneliness or pain. Maybe they cried for fear of the future, or fear of its absence. As a physician, I could even imagine that they cried because their strokes had affected emotive centers of their brain and that their sorrow was a function of disordered neurons and misdirected neural chemicals. The truth is, I don't know.

However I have developed a new theory. Over the years, as I have become a husband and father, I believe I have come to understand their sadness. I believe that they were mourning for the blessed mundane. I believe that both of them, steeped so solidly in the day to day of life, wept for the day to day, for the commonplace, for the small, seemingly inconsequential things that make up the brick and mortar of our lives.

50

From my own life, these are the things that seem deceptively small and commonplace. They are the times my wife and I share laughter in a disordered kitchen. They are bedtime stories and cups of milk in the middle of the night. They are diapers changed and bottles filled. They are afternoons when we sit on the floor and play a game, or pretend to be dragons while pre-school knights wave plastic swords. Sometimes, they are quiet moments of intense, speechless joy. These times are impossible to number every day: shared meals, shared dreams, wounds dressed, baths given, soft beds, good night embraces, drives to school in the morning, picking up from school in the afternoon, surprise lunches in the park and on and on.

I can look back and imagine some of the things my grandparents would have put in these categories, as well. They probably included meals prepared on Sunday, pony rides given to grandsons, new corn in the garden, the open window of a truck on a rural highway in the summer, the first look at a grandchild, or great-grandchild, ice-cream before bed, sleeping in a recliner, Sunday morning services and more than I can dream.

So I think that when grandma and grandpa cried, when their aged chests heaved with sorrow and we hugged them and wondered why, they were simply mourning for the mundane and common. In their nursing homes, for all of the well-meaning care they were given, nothing was as they remembered. The decades of common things that had surrounded them, the worlds of comfort and meaning they had established for themselves were no longer available to any of their senses. And our visits were poignant reminders of the wonder of simple, gentle things.

I imagine that when they were finally received into heavenly glory, God eased them gently into wonder. I doubt if they were met with his shining throne. I imagine it was into green grass and morning sun, and things of common wonder that their sorrow finally melted away.

Beautiful Girl

"Hey beautiful girl,"
he said to his frail bride
and touched her brittle hair,
white with bottle red.
Thin, shaking arms
held high like
"take me away,"
but she only moaned through
cracked lips.
But he, well, he
had clear eyes.
And touching his
beautiful girl, whom we
thought old, sick, doomed,
he saw her soft hair auburn,
her hands unwrinkled,
reaching up to hold him,
young full lips whispering,
"hey, handsome boy."

Time and Children

I'm in Atlanta for a conference as I write this. I drove just over two hours to get here and I'll be back home tomorrow. In spite of the short duration of my trip, my seven-year-old son Samuel cried and begged me not to leave home. I think that some of his feelings were based on fear. He has absorbed more than his share of the lessons of 9-11. He asks me, when I travel, if I will fly and if there are tall buildings. He has fears that no child should but that many around the world now do.

But there's more than his fear. There's the bond we share. We are connected in a way that I find difficult to describe. He has so much of me in him. He has my loves of words and images. Stories pull him into other worlds. He has my strengths and, sadly, my weaknesses. He has anxiety, which I passed to him as if fear were encoded on base pairs. He has my tendency to the emotional, to the sentimental. He is anthropomorphic, fearing that toys will feel lost or miss him. I remember that sentiment in childhood.

In his fear, however, Samuel teaches me a lesson. His lesson is that children understand the primacy of time. This is a thing that adults have forgotten. We believe that time management means wringing the most productivity (as defined by other grown-ups) out of every moment. We believe we have used our time well when, in one day we have worked our shift, read our journals, checked the news, scanned the web-sites of organizations important to us, eaten well and quickly, exercised briefly and played with our children for the allotted hour. Ah, time well spent.

But to a child, time is a paradox. It both exists and does not. It exists, perhaps, because they see that it is important to us. In this, they humor their parents, who have forgotten so much. They seem to understand that we function in a complex and somewhat false, labyrinth of days, hours, minutes and seconds. When we say, "in a minute", they know we mean an hour. And when we say "maybe next week", they sigh and realize that what we probably mean is never. Our earnest belief in time, our enslavement to its confines, is a punishment to our little ones. They suffer its privations. They endure our time management schemes. They look longingly for us to come to them with rich, unfettered hours to lavish on them like water to their parched hearts. What they receive is quality time, which means little time and less quality.

To a child, time is fluid. I imagine that children are much more connected to the mysteries of space-time than even the most astute physicist. Children believe that their birthdays will never come, even when they are only a week away. They feel certain that Christmas Eve is the longest night of the year. Time itself seems to slow down, as if God were halting it to give us our children, as children, for just a little longer and especially at the most sparkling moments of their lives.

And yet, time flies. Two hours of running and laughing pass in an instant. A vacation at the beach seems only one day long. "We just got here! We can't leave yet!" We think this is a ruse, a childish misrepresentation. But when they are lost in joy they are timeless. It must be painful when we snatch them back into the endless sweep of the hands of our damnable watches.

But the childhood twisting of time isn't limited to the hours of the day. It transcends that. Seth, my five-year-old, has assured me that he knew me when I was a little boy and that we played together. Who am I to say he didn't? Maybe he was sent to me for a while, a surprise playmate, in a park, whose mother was nowhere to be seen. Maybe in that capacity he could decide if he would come to live with me one day. It would explain why we play so well together. Maybe he chose me.

This transcendence also explains why children embrace eternity so easily. It makes sense. Why, with all the wonder and laughter and toys and pleasures of this life, should it all end so easily? Why should anyone be permanently separated? Why should deceased dogs and cats not come back to life again? Why shouldn't little boys and girls have a hope that if they lose their parents, they will be reunited in a place where no separations can ever occur? Sometimes the most simplistic theorems are the most critical.

Blessed man that I am! I have four small tutors in the mysteries of time. In their eyes I see the truth of my passage. I have spent too many years and too much time doing important things. I have studied and worked, gone to meetings and been on committees. I have read and networked and shaken hands and expressed how delighted I was to meet people who were important for this or that reason. And even though all of it was genuine, much of it is lost in the past. Names and projects will likely never be recovered. Meetings, which seemed so vital to my career or my department, are forgotten and their minutes shredded or burned.

But with my little ones, whether in play or reading, bathing or brushing teeth, praying or simply sitting on the couch, I am allowed access into a parallel universe where the rules are different. They slow down my time. They fend off aging. They stop my productivity, as I perceive it, and make me productive for them. And that productivity is best, born as it is of sheer delight in the holy moment, in the doing of things that feel good, that bring comfort, that make laughter. They help me to step away from time to experience the imperative of just being.

I've been looking around at the attendees of this conference. Distinguished persons surround me. I am only distinguished in my relative unimportance. I hear these great minds talk about their projects, their goals, their lives of writing reports and chairing organizations. I hear their lists of publications and read the complex titles after their names and I know that they have managed time well. I respect their drive. I just hope that it isn't too late for them to learn the lessons of time and timelessness, that only small children can teach.

DUI—Driving Un-Impeded

In my practice, I can safely say that alcohol causes more tragedy than just about anything and is a true bane of human existence. If it were invented today it would never pass FDA approval. I know that self-controlled individuals can use it responsibly. But let's face the fact that it causes people to do terrible things and its abuse has horrible consequences for users, their victims and society as a whole.

For instance, I've rarely seen a violent act in which someone wasn't intoxicated. Gun or knife, stick or fist, the very presence of alcohol heightens impulsiveness and lowers control. I've seen studies on alcohol related deaths from disease and car accidents, but I've never seen any that detailed the association between violence and alcohol. Nevertheless, I strongly suspect that the association exists. However, I don't want to address violence. That isn't my soapbox right now. Drunk driving is. And for the purpose of this article, I'd like to continue to refer to it in that manner. I think that "driving while intoxicated", or "driving under the influence" are simply too whitewashed, too kind. Put simply, put bluntly, I am tired of drunks driving cars. I am tired of taking care of them. And I am tired of seeing their victims.

Now let's get something straight right away. Drunk drivers aren't just decrepit old men in smelly coats and dilapidated pickups. Neither are they simply blue-collar laborers who spend their evenings in bars and swerve home after last call. Some drunks might be these things, but drunks are also middle and upper income men and women with nice careers, good jobs and expensive cars. They are professionals who think they can handle anything, go out for business dinners and then climb behind the wheel of their BMW, Lexus or Mercedes while impaired. Some are high school students who drive their parents' cars into trees, into other vehicles or over embankments. Quite a few are college students who somehow believe in their own immortality and invulnerability and therefore drink all night at parties. Then, they decide to go somewhere else with friends and find themselves sitting behind the wheel as their speech slurs, their vision blurs and they have to fight to stay awake. Party on.

It isn't just a Friday and Saturday night problem. In the Oconee Memorial Emergency Department we are seeing more and more drinking and driving on all of the other nights of the week. People used to exhibit a little embarrassment about such behavior. Now it seems to be perfectly acceptable. I find it entirely unacceptable.

The problem is current laws regarding DUI seem to be toothless, or at best ineffectively enforced. I have cared for many a drunk driver. And on the whole their behaviors are little altered by tickets, suspended licenses or jail terms. Many of them pay the fine, lose their license, don't worry about insurance (once their license is gone) and continue to drive the same vehicle they were driving when caught. Or they drive a friends' vehicle. Worse they consistently do it when they're drunk.

As for jail, it's a joke. They go to jail for the night and are out the next day. What about their conviction? Well here's a good example. I talked to a local deputy recently who told me of a case of DUI that he had taken to court. It was a seventh offense. The defendant was allowed to plea bargain down to a first offense. Boy that had to hurt! I don't doubt that the defendant celebrated with a few drinks that night.

If that story isn't good enough, I vividly remember a man I saw this year who had driven a tractor-trailer from Atlanta to our little corner of South Carolina. He pulled over at the truck stop and called EMS for help with his "chronic pain". I'm surprised he needed any help since he was seriously intoxicated with alcohol. Later, during the course of his care, he threatened to punch me. What did he get? One night, probably less than eight hours, in jail; he couldn't be prosecuted for DUI because responding officers didn't actually see him driving the truck (which was eventually driven away by "a friend"). . He was picked up again the next day for public intoxication. This isn't the fault of police. It's the fault of a system of laws that are failing to put fear in the hearts of lawbreakers.

South Carolina's highways are dangerous enough. I love my family more than words can ever begin to describe. So it's time to make them a little safer. And I have a proposition. It will take some guts. And it will take some intolerance of drunk driving. It might even take what modern pundits call "mean spiritedness". But here it is. Everyone convicted of drunk driving has his or her vehicle permanently confiscated by the state. No questions asked. They also lose their vehicle if they refuse the Breathalyzer or refuse to have a blood alcohol level drawn. The state impounds it and then sells it at auction. What if they still owe money on the vehicle? Not my problem. Can't drive to work? Get a ride. They should have thought of the consequences first. The legalities can surely be worked out. The owner must continue to pay on the vehicle. It simply belongs to the state, to do with it as the state wishes. What if it's someone else's vehicle? Then the state impounds it for a pre-set period of time, say one to two months and the person who was driving has to pay the car payments and pay for the owner's transportation to work. Now some will say that this is too harsh. That it imposes too great a financial burden. But what is really harsh is telling someone that their family member is critically injured or dead because of a drunk driver. And what about the financial burden of raising children alone, or the emotional burden of a lost child? Obviously, this is a fine much higher than existing ones. But it wouldn't take long for such a law to dramatically reduce drunk driving. You see, fines, jail and suspended licenses might be a joke, but confiscation of a $10,000 to $50,000 truck or car will get people's attention.

I'm not apologetic about this. We have to do something. The law needs more venom when it comes to drunk driving. The other thing that might help is a bit of good old-fashioned moralizing. People need to be ashamed of drunkenness again. It isn't cute anymore. It's life and death. I tell drunks that they could have killed my wife or my child on the road. I'm judgmental and mean when it comes to this issue. But I'm not unreasonable.

My plan doesn't punish alcohol manufacturers for crimes they don't commit. It doesn't punish auto manufacturers for failing to include safety equipment that wouldn't have mattered. It doesn't punish restaurants or bars for the irresponsible acts of their patrons. It hits the ones who do the crime, right where it hurts. Below the belt and in the wallet.

Breath Shepherd

I'm home tonight. Downstairs, in the stillness of this house, my wife and children sleep in warm beds. Walking through the house at night is wonderful to me; a symphony of breath, each person a separate instrument as they collectively breath in time to the metronome of life itself. It's interesting how something so common can move me so; but not surprising. How many years of my life have I devoted to breath? Or to its preservation? Airway, breathing, circulation. Always, breathing. And when I step, quietly, through the halls and doors of my darkened home, the rhythm of breathing fills me with secret joy and thanksgiving.

My wife Jan breaths heavily in her sleep, the breath of the tired laborer. Sixteen hours of parenting and the feather-bed receives her kindly, a worker who has earned her dreams. Samuel, my seven-year-old, breaths like he walks, with stealth. A child who with frightening silence, glides through the house and slips behind his victims to shout "gotcha!" He's my ninja. He loves the silence of the night, playing or watching movies, even driving in the car on trips. His breath is silent in the dark as still as he.

Seth, age five, snores his exuberance. His adenoids are too large and consequently, his sleep is interrupted by sputters and pauses of varying lengths. His sonorous breath as disarming as his smile; as loud as the energy with which he approaches play. I worry about his breath sometimes, but not too much. One day, those adenoids need to come out. When he is in the right position, he sometimes breaths quietly, a stocky angel, smelling vaguely of brownie.

Elijah, age two, is so quiet in his sleep that I often stop and put my hand on him. His breath moves his chest only slightly and sometimes I am compelled to put my hand by his mouth and nose to be reassured by the warm moist air that he softly exhales. Like his mother, he earns his sleep with intense play and more intense emotion through the long hours of light. Night is a relief for him and he crawls into bed with joy in his heart, asks to be covered in his soft blanket and drifts away to dreams that I probably could not fathom.

Elysa, age one year, breaths in a whisper of air. To quote Doctor Seuss, "Like the soft, soft whisper of a butterfly". Not a snore, I can hear it, but must listen closely. She is so bright and busy when she is awake, but in her sleep returns to the infancy so recently past. Sometimes I touch her too and occasionally wake her by accident in my zeal to ensure that oxygen is passing as it should into her lungs and into the blood that rushes beneath her pink-tinged alabaster skin. Her breath, like a wee cup of tea, is sweet and warm and moves in tiny volumes.

It isn't always so lovely and gentle. I recall nights when RSV infected my children and when their breathing was rapid and shallow. Jan and I sat many nights by wheezing, struggling children as we gave albuterol nebulizers and I wondered when to stop being their doctor, become their worried father and take them to the emergency department where my partners were working. The retraction of belly under ribs, the hollow cavity of the neck above the clavicles, these signs which we fear in children not our own are harbingers of abject terror when they appear in our own and cause otherwise sleepy nights to be filled with hour to hour, minute to minute uncertainty. And then, what a relief when no tubes need to be inserted into tracheas, when no ventilators cycle to replace the normal bellows of soft breath. What joy when sick children sleep with no threat that they may stop breathing and parents' minds can slip away to peace again.

More horrible still, I can recall times when my children choked on food eaten too fast. I remember with anxiety the look on Seth's face when the air would not move, when breath was far away, crippled by the imperative airway which was blocked with food. I remember how we smacked his back, how his face turned from crimson back to pink, and how thankful to God I was that he did not turn cyanotic and leave me. I remember my own times, waking with stridor from some bizarre combination of laryngitis and overly reactive lungs. I know that horrible sense that air, breath, would never come again. Breath the lovely becomes breath the priceless when it stops.

Small wonder that the word spirit is derived from the Latin, spiritus or breath. It seems, as our loved ones breathe, that life itself moves in and out of their bodies with perfect, cyclic regularity. That every cycle reproduces God's leaning over Adam; mere clay, and blowing divinity and animation into his inanimate shape.

Certainly, as doctors we see the analogy. The math is so simple. Breath equals life. No breath equals death. Spirit equals life, no spirit equals physical death. And we therefore spend our careers watching the rise and fall of fifty thousand chests, listening to the character and quality of the spiritus that moves in and out of every patient for whom breath has become difficult or in whom it may imminently cease.

So, there I am, a guardian of breath. Night watchman for the lives that are part of me, my family who sleep within my hearing, within my touch and sight. It is my most sacred duty to keep their breath safe. But next, to keep the breath of all of those patients who are my own. Breath guard, spiritus shepherd. I roam the night with fear and wonder, watching, listening and feeling for anything which might stop the very thing that enlivens us all.

And so, I think I'll go back downstairs and get back to the work that I love best and tip-toe between beds, listening, touching and watching as life itself floats through my family and my house for yet another night.

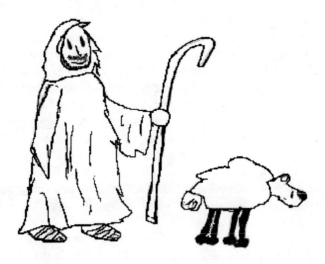

Quality of Life

Vacationing near a mountain lake in Tennessee, I watched as a young woman began the walk from her cabin to the pool where my children and I were playing. From a distance, I wasn't sure if she was old or young. She appeared heavy, wore a large hat and walked with a slightly awkward gait. It became clear as she drew closer she had been born with Down's Syndrome. She was probably in her late twenties or early thirties. She did not carry herself with grace or elegance. She was pale and her one-piece bathing suit plain, like those that grandmothers wear as they watch their grandchildren splash in the warm water on beaches at low tide

I was a little anxious. No family or friends accompanied her. She placed her towel on a lounge chair, sat down and faced the clear water. I wondered if she understood the danger and depth of the pool, as she sat relaxed near the deep end. My twin engines of worry, fatherhood and medical degree, began to make me anxious.

She moved to the edge of the pool and I fidgeted. Was she even supposed to be there? Was someone looking for her, concerned that she might come to harm? I quietly wondered these things as she slid into the water and began to glide across the pool with the even, silent strokes that I have always desired, but never accomplished. I don't believe that my jaw dropped, but I'm sure my eyes widened. I laughed to myself. She had spent years swimming; for all I knew she may have been a special Olympian. The water received and embraced her.

Her kicks were quiet and the cyclic movements of her arms made no splash on the surface. Her breathing was relaxed and measured and one might have assumed she was some aquatic creature, born and raised in the depths of the ocean. Like a seal, which seems out of place as it moves across the ice, her awkwardness dissolved in the water. The body which had seemed cumbersome on land became graceful and elegant the second she pushed away from the ladder. She was transformed before my eyes.

Too often, those of us with healthy bodies and minds imagine that our world, the one in which we individually dwell, is the best one. We believe, falsely, that imperfect lives are malformations and mutations that should never have occurred. It's easy to make sweeping statements about quality of life when our reference is the quality of our own. I saw in that young woman how easily I could be wrong and how wonderful it was to see the truth.

Sometimes I mistakenly think that God's destiny for certain groups is a thing that will begin when he makes them whole. That somehow, those with genetic anomalies or debilitating medical problems will simply have to suffer through and that we will suffer as we care for them until such time as they enter God's presence through death, or He returns to renew all life in the way originally intended.

But the truth is, I can't discern her quality of life. And I have no idea of God's destiny for her. I suspect that her quality of life is wonderful, if her swimming was any indication. And she lives, so God must have something in store for her destiny. Maybe we are only a discovery away from a chemical or genetic manipulation that will restore her and with a subtle flick of a biological switch, an activation of what someone thought was "junk DNA", transform her into something hidden in her chromosomes all along: world class athlete, intellectual giant, loving servant of mankind. Maybe not.

More likely, the ultimate value of her life is something that I will never know. God is under no obligation to explain these things to me. I think that he smiles as I ponder them, but that he will reveal them only in his good time. All I know is that in a few laps across the pool, that young woman showed me that every life has more value than I can ever begin to see and more wonder and potential than I can imagine. I hope I remember the lesson.

A Prayer For Us

Holy Father,

We go now into the uncertain
world to guard your children.
Where our hearts are hard,
soften them with your gentleness.
Where our minds are slow,
enliven them with your knowledge.
Where our hands are unsteady,
move them with your touch.
Where our bodies are weary,
stand by us, for you never sleep.
Help us for the sake of the sick,
and the wounded;
guide us for the sake of the dying,
and the grieving;
speak to us for the sake of the confused
and all who pass into our care.
Show us that our patients are your children,
and teach us to show them mercy as we
want mercy for our own.
And make us strong for the struggle each day.

Amen

Grandpa's Hands

It's still March. My hands, as usual, are cracked and bleeding from dry winter air and from the endless washing that comes with the practice of medicine. Lotion temporizes, but every day I work the same problem returns. By the time this is in print, in May, my hands will be fine. But for the duration of winter, the skin on my knuckles will crack, my fingertips will split and I'll look as if I reached into a box full of rabid raccoons, as nurses tsk, tsk and direct me to various hand cream regimens.

But I don't mind really. Because my hands connect me to my maternal grandfather, Wetzel Owens. Wetzel was a man whose image fills many of my childhood memories. Tall, thin, strong he was a truck driver and part time cowboy. The weather, combined with some unknown ancestry, had left his skin dark. In a checkered shirt, boots and hat, he looked like the trusty sidekick in a John Wayne western. He spoke of horses with a certainty and comfort8 that hinted that he might have been born in the wrong place and the wrong age.

Grandpa's hands were just like mine. All winter they split and cracked and his skin's vulnerability was all the worse for his natural tendency to hurt himself. So he was forever turning his wounded paws over and back, assessing each day's new damage and muttering to himself. I suppose his hands reflected that he was a man of activity, who was undeterred by elements or by pain. That's how I remember him.

When I remember him I also think of competence, usefulness, worth. Equally comfortable under the hood of his car or strapping a saddle to a paint pony, at ease in barn, warehouse, workshop or garden, he was so much that I never have been and never will be. I despise car repairs, I am marginally interested in horses and I can't nail two boards together without risking a smashed nail and a tragic, almost criminal misuse of wood.

So I find myself feeling incompetent by comparison. I have always felt inferior to the men who build houses or engines, who dismantle motors and pour concrete. I have spent my adult life measuring myself against those who work with their bodies and who seem to create order and structure out of nothing, using only strength, common sense, and calloused hands.

But then again there are my hands. They feel a little like Grandpa's. The ends split just like his did. The tops are leathery. A nurse, who recently started an IV on me, remarked that I must spend a lot of time outdoors, although I don't spend nearly enough. My hands have the superficial appearance of the hands of a workman. And maybe I am, in my own way.

When I was in college taking journalism classes my freshman year, I realized that I couldn't spend my entire life writing without having some skill to offer the world with my body, with my hands. I decided on medicine. Although I have begun to come full circle, I see what a blessing it was. Because the things I use my hands for bring me closer to the heart of humanity and give me the gift of stories.

The thing is, I not only chose medicine, but emergency medicine, which comes the closest to labor of any specialty. My hands split and hurt because I use them and wash them all day. When I come home my feet and back hurt, because I walk for miles per shift, sometimes move backboards, sometimes help lift people out of cars and wheelchairs. My eyes are blurry from focusing, my mind simply tired from thinking. My neck hurts from bending over wounds. My body feels spent at the end of the day.

Furthermore I mostly work third shift. How many other physicians describe their work schedule in such industrial terms? Do surgeons work "third shift"? Do internists or pediatricians? Instead, they take call. Only in emergency medicine do we divide our workday in the same manner as the laborers who come to us for care.

Even in financial terms, this specialty has parallels to other, non-medical vocations. Most of us make money based on patients seen or hours worked. We are paid for our productivity on the assembly line, in a way. Admittedly, for all of our complaints and imagined misery, we make vastly more than most people in the world. But the way we do it has a suggestion of factory work. Especially when held up to other specialists who make huge amounts for relatively short procedures.

When I think about all of this, I find my sandpaper hands reassuring. They not only tie me to my laboring, farming, mining ancestors, but they also connect me to the average men and women who come to me in this little Southern emergency room. Men and women who work like dogs for all their long lives, hands abused by textile mills, machine shops, shovels and tractors. It's good to relate to them, because their effort is honest. In caring for them I am a part of the productivity of the working world.

But my hands also remind me that Grandpa was proud of me while he walked the earth. I'm sure he still is. He knows that I work hard and care for his great-grandchildren well. He knows that my bleeding hands, while skilled in things different from his, are just as busy.

The Worst Lie is the One You Tell Yourself

Sometimes, a little brutal honesty is just what the doctor ordered. It hurts but then so does an antibiotic injection. Like the shot, honesty can make things better. So I think that we in emergency care, and every specialty, need to take a serious, honest look at what's going on in medicine and what the future holds. I'm no policy-maker; I'm only a clinician. But generals can't plan a battle without listening to the troops in the foxholes. And boys and girls it's ugly out here.

Volumes are rising, payment is falling, lawsuits from the feds and private sector lie around like punji sticks, waiting for us to step off of the narrow path we walk. We are faced with increased expectations, decreased resources and libraries of rules and regulations. But how did we get here? I think the answer is, dishonesty. We have lied to ourselves and have tried to create a reality that can't exist. As such, I have a little list of some of the lies we've been telling ourselves down the years. Here's a list of a few of the falsehoods we have assimilated and why I feel they are wrong.

1) "Medical care should be free and we should feel a little odd about wanting to be paid." This is an indoctrination that dates to our days in pre-med. It's a utopian ideal but it's pure fantasy. And it involves some "double-think". First, we bemoan the fact that our incomes are falling. We feel that we are unfairly compensated, especially since we bear the brunt of the un-funded mandate of EMTALA. Agreed. But then, we throw open the gates and invite more and more people to the party (many of whom will never pay anything) because of our guilt about the cost of health care combined with our deep-seated rescue fantasies. We then demonize insurance companies for raising prices and decreasing reimbursement to save money, knowing that economic reality dictates that the insured bear the burden of payment for the uninsured. All the while the Federal government tries to squeeze more blood out of the already anemic turnip of a broken system of entitlement via Medicaid and Medicare. The truth? Nothing that involves

68

someone else's labor, or material, can be free. It might be free to the patient who receives it, but it always costs someone.

2) "Everyone who comes to the ER has something that to them, is an emergency. These persons should always be treated with gentility and respect and reminded that we want them to come back as much as they feel necessary." Blah, Blah, Blah. Too much of what we see isn't even an emergency to the people who come! "I got bitten by a bug yesterday and it's red. What do you think it is?" (No trouble breathing, no dysphagia, no hives). "I think it was a bug, sir." This was not an emergency. This, my friends, was a life event. It includes normal menstrual cramps, sunburns, anger, break-ups and many other entities billed as emergencies. Drunkenness is also, for the most part, a life event. We need to remember this as police bring obviously intoxicated patients to be "checked out" before they can spend the night in the county hotel. Many of our patients don't belong in a family practice office, much less an emergency department. The sooner we address this firmly and politely, the less we will be overwhelmed by volume. Furthermore, a $5 co-payment on Medicaid visits would decrease a lot of the ridiculous things we see. "Five dollars for a bug bite? I can get some smokes for that! Forget it." You see, for all of our hand wringing about the uninsured and poor (and there are a lot of them I am delighted to help) many of the patients who use us for all their health care needs place zero value on our services, because Medicaid and EMTALA allow it to be priced at exactly that amount to the patient. Zero.

3) "We should be happy our volume is up!" That is, as sick patients wait 8 hours to be seen we should be happy that we are overwhelmed with non-paying patients and their life-events (see #2). The truth is, even sick patients who are paying customers often apologize to me for using the ED. Because they understand that care is important, that

the emergency department is for emergencies and that it costs real money. They pay for it. Patients who don't grasp this socioeconomic reality see no reason not to come and tie up the department because their friend had vaginal discharge and they thought it might be fun to check in for their "chest pain" and pregnancy test. Imagine how much this costs America! Also, too many people use the ED for entertainment. It's exciting to get mad at your girlfriend, "pass out" and have your buddies drag you out of the car at the ambulance entrance. Followed, of course, by the drama of cursing at nurses and doctors until said girlfriend returns and you both cry and hold each other.

4) "Everyone's pain is real and we should let the pain scale guide us in their treatment." Let me be blunt. The pain scale is one of the most useless therapeutic tools I have ever encountered. Everyone with any pain is now a ten, except for those who say, "No, it ain't a ten, it's a twenty!" From splinters to dog bites, laughing college students to grimacing "chronic pain" sufferers, everyone knows that they should say "ten." And of course, JCAHO, various pain organizations and our own ACEP have all been reminding us of how sloppy and uncaring we are when treating pain. Consequently, and I'm sure there's causality here, prescription drug abuse is sky-rocketing. Medicaid in South Carolina is imposing strict rules on prescribing Oxycontin. In several states, including Virginia and West Virginia, class action suits are being filed against Pharma (maker of Oxycontin) and against some of those who prescribed it. Why? Because of the large number of addicts created among patients who probably said, "It's a ten!". Here's the truth. We make a few pain management mistakes. But we generally know who hurts and who doesn't. It's part of being an emergency physician. See thousands of patients a year and you start to notice trends in behavior that signal pain. Furthermore every time that we cave in to the pain scale or any other politically correct

instrument in pain management, we create a nation of weak individuals, for whom the slightest discomfort requires the euphoria of narcotic analgesia. Pain isn't any fun. But much of it can be easily managed with over-the-counter medications or with nothing at all! I don't have any internal discord when I say, "That's what we call an ankle sprain and not a particularly bad one. Yeah, I'm sure it hurts but you don't need Lortab, Percocet, Mepergan, Oxycontin or any other prescription pain medicine for it. In a few days you'll be fine." Narcotic addiction isn't any fun either. It weakens our nation by causing enormous social and financial burdens due to medical care, accidents, crime and lost productivity.

5) "We make far too many medical errors. Just look at the Institute of Medicine Report! We have to do something to reduce the gross amount of errors we make and restore public confidence." First, the Institute of Medicine Report has been widely criticized. Despite that fact, continuous certification was thrust upon us as a specialty. Instead of defending our profession, we rolled over and whimpered like scalded dogs (that's a Southernism, by the way). When most large industries get bad press, they get good PR agencies. We could learn from that. I mean, I know we make mistakes. I've made them myself. But as a rule, I think we do an amazing job of not hurting people. Here's why. Take a look at the setting in which we practice one of the most risky types of medicine in America. In an emergency department, we see everyone, regardless of complaint and are expected to be knowledgeable in virtually every discipline of medical science. We move rapidly from paronychiae to cardiogenic shock, then back down the hall to sexual assault, on to HIV with fever and so on throughout our 8 to 12 hour shifts. And these are not patients we see regularly, with whom we have developed rapport. They are mostly strangers with whom we have a roughly two-hour window of opportunity to do the right

thing before they complain that their wait was too long. Many are on eight to ten medications. The potential for medication interactions is staggering. Into the mix, we are told, we should counsel about alcohol abuse, explore domestic violence issues, administer immunizations, cajole hesitant consultants to provide care for these people, find them rides home, ensure that their confidentiality is secure, even as we dictate and then give them a big, warm hug as they leave. The expectations are simply too immense for what we have set ourselves up to do. The truth? What we do is nothing short of miraculous.

6) "Everyone's welfare is our responsibility." Wrong. I do my job by attempting to care for the sick and injured. However, competent adults should be forced to be accountable for their own welfare. I'm their physician while they are in the emergency department, not their mommy. For instance, I'm not going out of my way to give you free samples when you smoke two packs of cigarettes a day. I'm not going to ask the nurses to make appointments for someone who has a home phone, cell phone and pager, but who says they just can't do it on their own. And I won't beg patients to stop using street drugs. We'll discuss it, but after a few failed attempts at rehab, I'm not sure what else I as a physician, or the system at large, should be expected to do. Bad decisions have bad consequences. The truth? When we take too much responsibility for patients, we make them weak. And we stress an already over-burdened system to the point of breaking.

7) "Health Care is a right". Ouch. This one gets into philosophy and theology. But in essence, it can't be true any more than any other thing that people need. People need houses, but if houses are a right, then builders have to work for free. And when that happens, it's back to thatch huts. It's that simple. Rights have to be non-tangible; things that can't be touched. The right to free speech, the

72

right to freedom of religion, these are rights that do not require the action of others, only the inaction. That is, they exist so long as no one interferes with them. Services and tangibles are different. If food were a right, then the faint profit margin of grocers would fade to negative numbers and grocery stores would only exist as subsidized government institutions. You could get the basics, like bad bread in Soviet Russia, but gourmet coffee and fresh salmon would be hard to come by. Health care, economically, can't really be a right without the ultimate financial devastation of socialized care. Just watch what happens when the Medicare prescription drug benefit (read "right") starts. It will be a lesson for us all.

So that's my list. It's obviously only partial. I'm certain I've missed some big ones. I may seem like an evil, right-wing curmudgeon. But that isn't true. I'm not evil. I care about patients and about the welfare of the country at large. I just think that improvements require that we face reality. It's difficult, but it's liberating. In the end the profession will only benefit as we remove the blinders and see the light.

Hope for my Child's Disease

I hate to be my children's physician. I do it with reservations. I'll treat the sore throat. I'll give breathing treatments for the wheezing. But sometimes I reach uncomfortable territory. On March 22, 2002, my hand was forced when my 5-year-old, Seth, began drinking like he had just come in from the desert. He had Scarlet Fever. I assumed he was drinking because his throat was sore. But when he said it wasn't and refilled his cup over and over. I knew it was time to look further. I was afraid of the obvious. That he had diabetes. So we went to the ED where I work and checked his glucose. It was 608, a number I won't forget. He looked at me confused, uncertain why people he barely knew were sticking his fingers, then drawing his blood. He was incredibly brave but I imagine he believed it was temporary. That he would go home and life would be back to normal. That's what I kept hoping and praying. That's what I continue to hope and pray as we attempt to make his transition to diabetes as smooth as possible.

Diabetes sucks. There's no other way to put it. I hate everything about it, just as I'm sure Seth hates everything he so far understands about it. We have all cared for patients whose bodies have been decimated by the assault of glucose and the total retreat of their pancreas. It's inane that a molecule so tiny can take a body and destroy it. But it's reality. And so I teeter back and forth, worried one day that he will have profound hypoglycemia; the next day that he will have poorly controlled sugars and develop retinopathy and renal failure. I need something like insulin to smooth my worry curve throughout the day. My wife Jan is keeping me calm. She handles stress with organization. My coping skills amount to enormous amounts of irrational worry. Seth, thanks to the prayers of many, has been heroic in his adjustment.

But trouble always has a lesson and in this case, more than one. As a physician I've learned a lot from this terrible time. And I think one of the most useful things I've learned is the importance of genuine compassion, having recently received so much of it. I thought I learned it from my kidney stone, or from the time Samuel, then age 2, was hospitalized with RSV as his chest struggled to move air in and out. I

74

thought I learned it from all of the fevers and vomiting and every other illness that Jan and I have faced over untold sleepless nights with four children. But apparently I didn't know much. For now, with a child facing a lifelong medical condition, I see more clearly the immense pain of parents whose children suffer. It is likely the worst pain a parent can experience.

I remember meeting many parents of sick children down the years with diseases both acute and chronic. I know there were times when I couldn't understand their hostility and frustration. I know that I tried to be the rational doctor and explain why they shouldn't worry. Or explain that I was sorry, but that there really wasn't anything else we could do in the emergency department. I remember thinking that they were so difficult and that I couldn't imagine being a pediatrician. You know the saying from medical school: "The kids are great, it's the parents that are tough!" I know why the parents are tough. The parents are tough, quite often, because the parents are scared to death.

What the parents see is their hope, their dream, their heart of hearts lying in a hospital bed suffering from a disease or infection, that is often invisible. Their parents see their children being molested and abused by bacteria, or viruses, or glucose or by the treasonous betrayal of their own DNA turned against them. What their parents cannot see is any way to stop it. If a person or animal were attacking their children, they would fight with their own lives. If it were a fire, they would cover their child with a blanket and run to the door. If their child were drowning they would swim to them and pull them to safety. But when their children are ill, parents are worse than powerless. They stand by the bed and stroke their children's hair; they fill hospital rooms with stuffed animals; and they wander the halls, wishing for normality and blaming themselves, either for being useless to take away the pain or for the imagined belief that they caused their child's condition.

What they need, in super-therapeutic doses, is compassion. They need for someone to listen as they tell the story over and over. They need to sit with someone who understands their fear and is willing to help them shoulder it for a while. In the Sermon on the Mount, Christ said we are to "mourn with those who mourn". Unfortunately, it's much easier once we have suffered a bit ourselves. It's easier to know the fear of a parent when one has become a parent. I didn't understand this until my children were born. And my grasp of compassion grew exponentially after March 22.

But compassion is only part of the equation. Because parents of sick and injured children need hope as well. It's so easy for us, with scientific clarity, to say that family members need to know the truth, the harsh reality. The statistics on mortality and morbidity from the condition their little one is enduring. And even while this may be true, it isn't the whole truth. At least in the beginning as parents are faced with the enormity of what life has dealt them, we need to offer some hope; even hope in the miraculous is better than no hope at all. And it isn't a lie. We have all seen things happen in medicine that defy science. It's OK to offer that hope, however fragile or fleeting.

One of the most wonderful things that happened to our family has been the outpouring of compassion and hope from friends, family and people involved with Seth's care. Two of our nurses have children who were diagnosed this year with juvenile onset diabetes. They have been a wealth of information. In the beginning, when I was hardest hit, my partners offered me this treasure: "Maybe this is a temporary inflammation of his pancreas related to the Strep! I'm sure I've read about that!" And the endocrinologist we are seeing said to us: "Frankly, I expect a cure inside twenty years. The trick for now is to keep Seth from having too many lows or highs and keep his Hemoglobin A1C at a good level. That way we protect him from complications and keep him healthy until the cure comes along!" The cure! Words I needed desperately to hear and believe.

Compassion and hope go hand in hand. I feel more of both these days. Compassion for my own child. Compassion for the parents of children who are ill. And I have special compassion for those children whose diseases have no cure and whose parents hope chiefly in unlikely statistics and the mercy of Heaven.

I'm fortunate. My child has a disease for which a cure is almost tangible. He was born in a time when diabetes is not the worst disease imaginable. I have hope in the brilliance of scientists, hope in the fortitude of my child, hope that his mother and I can keep his world as normal as possible and hope in the grace of his Creator.

I have another hope. I hope that those who read this will not face this trial. That everyone's insights can come from reflection rather than experience. Because most of all, if I could change it, I would take Seth's disease away and give it to myself. Because I'd rather learn about hope and compassion through my own discomfort than through his.

The Mysteries of the Night

When I wrote this, I was hoping to write something personal and touching that would help my brothers and sisters to practice with more compassion and care. I spent a few nights pounding the keys trying to get meaning out of a family experience involving health care. But then a strange thing happened. I worked a run of weekend nights and I decided it would make more sense to make fun of patients. So compassion, care, hope and meaning will have to wait. Besides, that article needs to age a bit. But sarcasm, irony and venom I have in excess.

The thing is, nights in general are a time of weirdness. They can be times of wonder and fascination. They can be times when we save lives and make obscure diagnoses. But mainly, in the emergency department, nights are times of the bizarre and inexplicable. I realize that some patients who use the ER at night are actually quite ill, or they wouldn't be there. For some, however, it's just the opposite. They wouldn't come out in the day if you offered them free lottery tickets and a carton of Marlboroughs. As a physician who works a lot of nights, I have remarked before that these persons, who populate my workplace from 2300 to 0700, are "my people". And it's true. I have developed an ability to work with them and understand them. I expect to smell alcohol, be asked if it's OK to go smoke before admission to the ICU, and sew up lacerations induced by various blunt and sharp objects. I'm OK with that. In fact, when I work days or evenings and everyone is sober, I feel out of my element. As such, I feel my people owe me a little something. And since money doesn't seem to be one of those things, they owe me material for writing. They owe me their stories, happy or tragic. And they owe me their humor. Or whatever humor I can develop from the events and complaints that bring them to see me when I would much rather be reclining in the lounge watching CMT.

I have compiled a short list of night shift mysteries. I've always loved the odd, the paranormal. The sort of thing I used to watch Leonard Nimoy talk about on the show "In Search Of". Today, I am in search of "mysteries of the emergency room." And there are a bunch.

These can be divided into three general sub-categories: medical, social and disorders of reality.

Beginning in the medical category, ask any patient at night what they were doing when their symptoms began. Any symptom, mind you, from chest pain to vaginal discharge. The answer? Watching TV. I used to puzzle over this. But it makes perfect sense. Either TV is profoundly unhealthy, which I suspect is true having watched the networks recently, or people watch so much of it that whatever happens is statistically most likely to occur while the tube is glowing in their pale faces.

Next, why does everyone have a relative who had a similar illness/complaint and who died a death so horrible and bizarre the story should have appeared on national headlines? "Well sure you say it ain't my appendix, but my cousin Jimbo, his appendix up and exploded (his wife heard it) and he died like a dog. Only thing he had was a runny nose." Or this perennial favorite: "I know little Bobby is only six years old, but when he said his chest was hurting, I realized that his great-grandfather died of a heart attack. I thought it was better safe than sorry and brought him down to get him checked out." Family history, it appears, is much more critical than we ever realized.

This weekend I had a run of abdominal pain patients. The mystery was this: how can so many people suddenly have abdominal pain at exactly the same time and with symptoms so similar that I can't tell any of the ten of them apart? Did the abdominal pain angel pass over? Fortunately, after finding virtually nothing objective on any of them, I settled back into the reality of ambiguity. This is a skill learned after many years, critical for working nights, that enables me to say with perfect comfort; "I have absolutely no idea what's wrong with you, sir. But I feel quite certain you won't die from it. At least not tonight."

Now, what marketing genius decided that every octogenarian needed to have a blood pressure cuff at home? There's a mystery worth solving. "Doc, I was watching TV (see?) and felt kind of funny. My blood pressure was 130/80. But I took it again and it was 150/90. And I got worried and took it again and it was 180/100, so I just called 911!" I should be able to call a representative of the company that manufactured the home cuff and congratulate him or her, each time, on the flawless operation of their device.

Medical mysteries are obviously difficult. But in the emergency department, we face hopeless mazes of social problems. In fact, much that is medical begins as social. Thus, social mysteries abound. Like this one: why are people who live their lives jobless, on Medicaid and welfare, so frequently and frighteningly obese? More simply, where else in the world are poor people consuming dangerous amounts of food? Images of famine and poverty in remote Africa seldom feature entire villages waddling about in search of "all-you-can-eat" restaurants and oversized spandex pants. Maybe lions eat them because they're slow. Lions: there's an idea for the obesity epidemic.

Of course, some social mysteries are not so mysterious. They're simply deception. For example: why does the chronic back pain patient, on disability and hourly narcotics, need a work excuse for the next day when his chart says "unemployed"? I have a friend who investigates disability fraud. I think he's a patriot.

Back to the young patient population. Why is it that every drunk, female college student with vomit for hair gel has a mouthy friend who says, "I think someone slipped her a pill. She drinks all the time and she's never like this! Are you going to check her for drugs? My dad is a doctor and he said you should check her!" Stunned, I stare at her and say "let's wait till we see what her blood alcohol is." I love going back to tell them that little Cassie has an alcohol level of 250 being processed through her 105 pound body. Drugs? Not so much.

Of course, that one crosses the boundary into the next category, the disorder of reality perception. This occurs when patients and other health care workers can't grasp reality. I love this exchange:

"So Miss Hall, could you be pregnant?"

"Absolutely not."

"Are you sexually active?"

"Yes."

"With a man?"

"Yes."

"Do you use birth control of any sort?"

"No."

"So, you could be pregnant."

"No, I couldn't."

"Do you have ovaries, a uterus and monthly cycles?"

"Of course."

"Has your sexual partner had a vasectomy or tragic chainsaw accident?"

"No."

"Then, miss, you could be pregnant!"

"No, I couldn't".

Be careful. This sort of exchange could cause you to be sucked into the black hole of ignorance forever.

Another conundrum I experienced this weekend is this: "I woke up at 2 AM all weak and tired." And? Whenever I wake up in the middle of the night I feel week and tired. I feel weak and tired when people tell me they're weak and tired. That's called fatigue. It is most properly treated with an experimental drug called sleep.

A similar mystery; Why is it that nursing home staff members feel compelled to send 95-year-old men and women to the emergency department, by ambulance, for weakness. These are people whose aerobic workout consists of watching someone else work a puzzle. They have Alzheimer's. They have no more muscle mass than a KFC drumstick. Of course they're weak. If I live to be old and infirm, I'll probably be weak too. Heck, I feel weak right now.

And what list of mysteries, especially those of reality perception, would be complete without the "no one was driving the car" story. Six people all ejected, all intoxicated, but apparently being driven down the road by the ghost of Elvis Presley. It's less of a medical mystery than a macabre thriller.

I realize that my patients are more complex than I can ever imagine. I also realize that some of the things I think are crazy are probably real problems that come in under my radar. But most of them aren't. They're just a function of the weirdness that is third shift in the emergency department. I know that this is a partial list. It's so partial, in fact, that I plan to continue compiling these oddities and write a periodic update. It should be easy unless I mysteriously hit the lottery and stop seeing mysterious patients altogether.

Betrayed by my Slacks

Outsourcing has finally hit home with me. Apparently, all the new slacks I attempt to buy have been outsourced to a location where a size 34 waist is actually about a size 28. What I want is my pants outsourced to a place where size 34 is equivalent to size 38. My home state of West Virginia comes to mind. That way I'll feel more comfortable without being reminded of the terrible reality that I eat too much. Of course, the reality was first revealed to me by my dear wife, who pinched my side and said, "Look, you have love handles, that's so sweet!"

The problem is multi-factorial. First, I was trying a new fitness plan through the winter. I called it "Dr. Leap's eat whatever you like and try not to exert yourself plan." It didn't work out too well. Not only did I gain wait, but now a game of hide and seek with the kids leaves me feeling out of breath. So much for my dreams of diet plan fame.

The other problem is that I am an emergency physician by trade. Which means that my schedule is erratic, I sleep poorly and eat too much drive through food. Co-workers in the hospital know I have arrived at work when they see the MacDonald's bag parked on the desk, along side the large sweet tea. Sometimes the bag contains a salad, so I'm not entirely evil. Sometimes I order a "filet-o-fish" just to annoy our unit secretary with the smell. Sometimes I order a Big-Mac, just to flirt with my own mortality.

MacDonald's always catches the heat in the national debates on obesity and healthy lifestyles, but there are other culprits. I love Wendy's chicken nuggets, sandwiches from Chic-fil-a, fish from Captain-D's and assorted other goodies that make health-food advocates have sweaty nightmares.

Fortunately, I've recognized the error of my ways. I'm eating less junk, exercising more and realizing that my inactivity/free-range grazing ways simply won't work if I want to stay healthy and active for my wife and children. Furthermore, it just feels better to be in shape. At least I remember that it felt good. So hopefully, I'll be slimmer as summer comes.

But one thing is certain. My fitness is my own responsibility. That's a tough pill to swallow nowadays. Everyone wants their weight problems to be the result of some dark industry plot to addict the world to breakfast biscuits, or even better, some genetic flaw that makes their obesity a disease rather than a lifestyle problem.

Admittedly, the fast food industry doesn't make it easy. They know how to make food taste good. Having eaten some low-carb pasta recently, I can say with utter clarity that a Taco-Bell beef burrito leaves low-carb pasta in the dust. Humans like things that taste good and fat adds taste. But I can't accept the notion that the fast food industry has done anything especially sinister. They're just doing what businesses do. That is, sell what the people want. If no one bought their product, they'd change.

Of course, some people find it harder to resist the overwhelming "yumminess" of fast food. We all have our weaknesses. I can't stop drinking tea despite two kidney stones. But at least I know that the next time I feel the sensation of a saber sticking in my back, it will be my fault, not Lipton's. It's the same for fast food. Our cars are not programmed to pull into the drive through.

Now I do know that there are those with medical conditions that make weight gain almost inevitable and weight loss next to impossible. But these are the minority. Most of us who gain weight in varying degrees do it because we just can't manage to limit the amount, or type, of food that we eat. And many who attribute their weight to genes simply were born into families that taught them to love the wrong foods in the wrong amounts and who failed to mention the word "exercise".

But no matter what factors contribute, obesity remains an American tragedy. It manifests itself in disease, dysfunction, depression and self-image horrors. And in the end, only one thing can save the majority of us from our dietary habits. That thing is the exercise of free will in the closing of our mouths. And neither lawsuits nor government intervention can close them for us.

HIPAA: Madness Legislated

The hospital risk manager spoke to our group recently. Her concern was with the privacy aspects of the HIPAA legislation. Everyone who sees a health care provider has heard of this by now. It stands for Health Care Insurance Portability and Accountability Act. While it concerns keeping insurance while changing jobs, one of its biggest concerns is the confidentiality of personal medical information. And if our little corner of the world is any indication, hospital workers from cook to cardiologist and everyone in between are being frantically educated in ways to avoid violating the confidentiality of patients.

Now I admit, confidentiality is important. Much like the feeling we get when checking out in the grocery store and hearing, "Price check on Fungex foot cream!", no one wants to smile nervously at the patient across the open curtain as the nurse says, "Wow, that's the worst herpes I've ever seen!"

But in these days of federal regulations that fall like rain in Seattle, HIPAA is being taken a bit too far. For instance, our well-meaning risk manager said, "I'll be walking around, and if I can hear you dictating, I'm going to tell you!" Even more insane, our unit secretary recently had a gall-bladder scan for severe abdominal pain. The hospital informed all secretaries that looking up their own lab or x-ray data was a violation of HIPAA, and if the computer snitches found out it had happened, jobs would be lost. The reasoning? Patients can't look up their information, why should you look up yours?

It isn't just the emergency room. A friend, who is a family doctor in a practice with one other MD and one physician's assistant, informed me that it would cost his office $30,000 to become HIPAA compliant and that they could no longer use sign-in sheets at the front window. Oh no! Someone might know that other people get sick too!

It has even been suggested to us that we stop using names to call patients from the waiting room, but rather, use animal code names. Of course, who wants to be Mr. Weasel or Mrs. Cow?

In light of this rollicking madness, which makes even EMTALA and the pain scale look like old friends, I have developed some policy suggestions:

When patients check in to the emergency department, they will be issued a code number. But because anonymity can't be ensured simply by not calling names and because we are visually oriented creatures, a plastic Halloween mask will be issued to all patients, as well as any family concerned that their confidentiality might be violated. Because triage, registration, nursing and physician staff might recognize patients, we will all wear blindfolds and learn to examine patients without the aid of our eyes. Of course, this could raise charges of inappropriate physical contact, but hey, at least we won't know who we inappropriately touched! It will be just like that Nirvana concert you went to back in college!

To ensure that patients do not use other physical clues to identify one another, individual waiting cubicles will be assigned to all patients. Nursing staff will bring patients into the emergency department by calling only the code number. To avoid any connection between code names and real names all registration staff will be injected with small doses of sedatives at 30-minute intervals to induce partial amnesia.

Once in the emergency department patients will be issued voice-scrambling devices like they use on television when interviewing Mafia informants. Doctors and nurses who wish to remain incognito will also have the option of using these devices and will be allowed to use code names for themselves. These code names will be approved by a consortium of members from the hospital ethics committee, the risk management office and the local branch of the ACLU. (So as not to offend).

Patients who require medications during computer malfunction will receive them by nurses directed to the bedside by doctors in a game of "Hot/cold", so that no names will be compromised. (You know, hot, hotter, no not there, cold, colder, warm, etc.). Difficult and dangerous due to the blindfolds, but very, very private.

Patients will be discharged and asked to mail their mask back to the emergency department, so that no one can see them leaving the hospital, and thereby assume that they have some social disease, mental problem or anything else which might make people say things like, "Hey Joe! Saw you leaving the hospital the other day!", which could obviously result in multi-million dollar jury settlements.

On the other hand, we could just issue code names at birth, known only to the government. The government, as in the case of the IRS, would obviously keep these codes inviolate and would never in a million years let them leak, or use them for untoward purposes.

Oh yeah and Grouch Marx glasses, with the big nose and mustache. If we all wore those, the world would be a much more private place.

Back to reality. Everyone, I mean everyone, gets sick and goes to the doctor or hospital. This isn't shameful and it isn't evil. It's reality. We shouldn't state chief complaints or diagnoses in front of other people and we shouldn't lay out records for the public to view. Isn't that an easier set of rules to follow? I guess the problem is, it would make so much sense that it could never happen.

So this is XQk-473z, MD signing off. See you around privacy rangers!

Why Emergency Departments Close

Across America there is a growing crisis in emergency care. Like fire, police and EMS it is generally taken for granted that emergency health care is available. However, while those entities are publicly funded (except for private or volunteer services), emergency care in hospitals is not. This reality is becoming all too clear in places like West Virginia, Florida and California where emergency departments, even those with trauma centers, are closing because financial concerns are making their operations impossible.

This was highlighted in a feature piece in USA Today entitled "ER conditions: Critical." Five reasons were suggested for ER overcrowding: "More and sicker patients in ERs; fewer hospitals, ERs and beds; nursing cutbacks and shortages; more treatment in the ER (i.e., new drugs and technology); and lack of access to other health care."

Now, there is no question in my mind that all of these contribute to ER overuse and fiscal difficulties. Actually, all of these things are true to a greater or lesser extent because emergency medicine has created a unique niche for itself in the medical milieu of America. It has made itself indispensable. And in so doing, it has become the default safety net for American health care. No one recognizes this more clearly than the federal government. They realize that health care in America is essentially impossible for them to fund. But they have an escape button through a law enacted in 1986, entitled EMTALA. This stands for the Emergency Medical Treatment and Active Labor Act. The spirit of the law is good. It prevents a physician or hospital from transferring or denying care to any patient with a medical emergency, or active labor, based on financial imperatives. (At least until that patient has been evaluated and stabilized). In the days before the law, unstable patients were too often loaded into ambulances and sent from private hospitals to public because they couldn't pay. This is called financial screening and EMTALA forbids it for any facility that accepts Medicare, on pain of harsh fines and potential imprisonment. But the reality of the law is closing emergency departments and hospitals across the land. Because it doesn't provide any money for the mandate it creates.

Actually the law allows an emergency department to medically screen a patient to make sure that they don't have a life or limb threatening illness (or labor), and then refer non-emergent patients elsewhere for further care. But screening exams have been anything up to and including surgery. So any emergency physician or facility with legal sense will simply accept the potential loss of money in the interest of avoiding litigation with the patient and with the Department of Justice (and the far greater loss of money that would entail).

Am I just another whining doctor who wants more money? No, I just want to point out another reason to the causes of ER closings and overcrowding. It is a reason seldom discussed in academic and government circles, because in the parlance of political correctness it is probably considered "mean spirited". But sometimes the truth hurts, so here goes. Many patients abuse ERs, even if they've never heard of EMTALA, because they understand that they can't be turned away or asked to pay up front. And when patients abuse ERs, the cost of care and the time spent waiting goes up for everyone.

At the hospital where I work, we have one patient who is sweet as glazed doughnuts. But, in the last 10 years, she has been seen some 400 times. No, that's not an extra zero. She knows, for all of her sweetness, that we can't turn her away. And her complaints, though rooted in anxiety, are usually of chest pain or shortness of breath. We have to take her seriously. She has insurance, though I swear I don't know how she keeps it. So it isn't just the money. It's the fact that each of those visits requires physician and nursing time. Each visit uses resources. And each evaluation takes time away from other patients and prolongs their care. Also, without any doubt, her care drives up the premiums for others with her insurance plan.

She's one of the nice ones. There are plenty of others. There are young women who miss their period and come to the ER for pregnancy tests. (And home tests don't cost more than the two packs of cigarettes they smoke each day, so that excuse won't wash). There are some whose friends or family members are inpatients or ER patients and who sign in saying, "I was here anyway, thought I'd get checked out too". For many of these the real emergency is boredom.

And there are some with repetitive illnesses that are purely of their own creation, like those patients whose alcohol abuse results in recurring injuries from car accidents or fights. Or the ones who are addicted to narcotics and go from ER to ER shopping for unsuspecting caregivers to give them another hit. There are those who, in spite of having emphysema or recent bypass surgery, smoke 2-3 packs of cigarettes each day. They know that they can always call the ambulance and come to the ER to be snatched from the jaws of death yet again and never feel the full financial or social impact of their actions.

Whatever business you may be in, imagine how the cost to your clients and the quality of your service would change if you were compelled by federal law to do it all, or give it all for free just for the asking. Imagine how long your business would stay open. Imagine how the clientele would use your time. This strikes at the real heart of the problem with emergency care in America. And until we get a handle on this harsh reality, the unfunded safety net is going to get mighty worn. And one day, when you or I fall into it, it will break. And when it does, the consequences will be tragic.

I Want to Eat Your Head

Storming into the emergency department, one of the physicians on staff at our hospital held his hands out as if asking a question, then launched into a series of angry accusations directed at me. Next, in his excellent but slightly accented English, he proclaimed "When I see your face in my mind today, I want to swallow your head!" Swallow my head? I've been threatened before. You know the standard "I know where you live and I'm going to kill you", or the more mundane "You'll hear from my lawyer". These were from patients. I expect them to threaten me. But I can't ever remember hearing anything quite like this from a fellow physician. And frankly, my head isn't that small.

It all stemmed from an interaction the night before that turned out badly in the light of day. You know how it goes. I think a patient should be cared for one way, the consultant doesn't. Looking back, I probably could have handled it differently. If I had, I could have allowed my fellow staff member to avoid the frustration of what I can only assume is a failure of the English language to describe something very clearly understood in his native tongue. But disagreements and conflicts happen. And sometimes someone just wants to swallow your head.

I hate conflict. I always have. I don't like to yell or argue with anyone. Not with my children, not with my wife, not with my parents and certainly not with my fellow physicians. Arguments make my muscles quiver and my stomach shake. They rob me of my ability to say anything witty or urbane. They leave me saying things like, "fine" or "whatever". The sort of things that angry teenagers say.

On the other hand, even at my worst, I don't plunge into screaming tirades or break innocent, inanimate objects. I don't go home and pace or write angry letters. Occasionally I fall back on the well-entrenched passive aggression that I learned from my family down the years. Generally, I simply let conflict go when I leave for home.

But this conflict was different. This whole "head swallowing" thing actually made me mad. I felt testosterone surge through my body, resulting in a sort of terrible serenity. And so, when my sparring partner explained for a second time that he wanted to consume my cranium, I responded more like a South Carolina redneck than a professional. "Do we need to take this to the parking lot?" Did I really say that? Did I really respond to a professional conflict like a drunken college student on Saturday night? Yep, I really did.

Now mind you, I'm telling all of this as a sort of confession. I'm not proud that I said it. Looking back, I seem to recall that a number of nurses stopped what they were doing and looked around about the time those words came out of my lips. Of course, they had been looking obliquely at the whole thing for the 30 minutes or so that it dragged on. They knew that my head was in danger of being digested. They just didn't expect me to counter the gracious offer of consumption with my own offer of a roll around the asphalt. I think I was feeling anger because I didn't believe I was entirely in the wrong and also because I had been awake all night, so that my inner control mechanisms were off-line.

Truthfully, I didn't really mean it. But when someone twice, in one loud conversation, offers to digest your calvarium, it starts to sound serious. I think that saying "do you want to go to the parking lot" was kind of a distraction. I think it surprised my colleague, who finally laughed in the midst of a tirade that would have made an auctioneer proud. "No, No!" He laughed again. The nearest nurse seemed to breathe a sigh of relief. Fortunately, we didn't go to the parking lot. We just stood there and kept yelling at each other. Finally, it all cooled down. I apologized for not handling things differently. He apologized too. We shook hands, we miraculously stopped talking and I ended the shift with my head still attached to my body. I left town for the weekend soon after and spent several days feeling badly. I hope that he and I can come to some sort of amicable working relationship from now on. I think I may have to apologize again when I go back home and see him. Even now, I'm haunted by my distaste for conflict.

Like every physician, I've had my share of battles. I've been treated like a simpleton by an out of town Ob-gyn who wanted me to send his patient to him immediately so he could treat her reflux, when she was actually suffering from HELLP Syndrome. I've been lectured on the necessity of ordering liver function tests on a schizophrenic patient before sending her to a psychiatric hospital. Over the years I have been slyly insulted, openly insulted, talked down to and ignored. I've had degrading conversations with sarcastic physicians and been treated like a hick by physicians at nearby tertiary care centers. I guess it comes with the turf.

In the process of such treatments, I have expressed my anger a few other times. I once told someone they should move out of our area and practice somewhere else if they didn't want to take care of patients. I think, in a minor flurry of "negative energy", that I asked a physician if he had actually gone to medical school. I know that I occasionally slam down phones. I offered to get a portable phone for a patient so that he could call his attorney, as he threatened he would, at 3:00 AM. I could go on, but then no one would hire me if I ever needed another job. I have never struck anyone in anger (not since 5th grade, and Mike was asking for it). I have not, since residency, used profanity toward a patient. (I was suffering from an unfortunate moral lapse that night in Indianapolis). And I have never threatened a patient or staff member. All in all, anger really isn't a problem for me.

Unfortunately conflict is a problem for all of us. Because somewhere along the line, physicians seem to learn that if you're angry enough, then you can say whatever you want to another physician or to a nurse. I hear stories. Stories of screaming fits, stories of instruments thrown down, clipboards flung across rooms. I hear stories of nurses left in tears, of doctors cursed thoroughly by other doctors. I have never understood any of this, except to say that the way in which we deal with our anger reflects a great deal about our professionalism, but even more about our maturity. My children throw tantrums sometimes. My daughter, 2 1/2 years old, is an artist and rage is her medium. I expect it from her. I have learned that ignoring her is the deepest cut and usually ends her outbursts. I guess ignoring some of the tantrums we see in hospitals may be the best tack as well.

I can't imagine working in a place where such anger was commonplace. I work in a community hospital and truly unpleasant encounters are unusual. We live near each other. Some of our kids go to school together. We need one another professionally and socially. Feuds, though they still occur, are generally impractical. And fits of rage make the rounds in about two hours. By the time I came back to work the day after my little "incident", people were asking me "did you almost get into a fight?" They all know me well enough to realize that I wouldn't have gotten into a fight. But just the thought made a good story. And by now, it's one that does not make me proud. It does make me laugh though, that someone might say, "that doctor Leap is a little bit crazy". After all, the night shift doctor needs that sort of publicity sometimes.

In the end it was a lesson to me. It was several lessons actually. The first was that most conflicts can be pre-empted before they need to be resolved. And as a physician, it's my job to keep things moving calmly and smoothly for the sake of everyone. I need to avoid unnecessary battles for the sake of the patients who need me and also for the physicians who are just as tired and frustrated as I am. The second lesson was that sometimes my indignation is actually righteous. It isn't wrong to stand for what I believe, as long as I'm willing, when the smoke clears, to accept that I might also have been wrong. And the third is that when someone threatens to eat part of your body, they generally don't mean it. I think.

Angelic Visitations

You just never know when Toni will show up. It may be morning, noon or after midnight. It may be because she really thinks she's dying, or simply to deliver the day-old doughnuts that she gives us as an expression of gratitude. She has no established pattern. When the triage light goes off and the nurse or medic brings a chart back while rolling their eyes, you can bet it's Toni. She's a fixture at our hospital. In fact, she has had over 800 visits to our emergency department since the early 1990's. She's almost like staff.

Her presentation has little variance. It usually involves clutching her chest, head hung down, too tight satin blouse half opened, black or red wig askew, teetering on high heels two sizes smaller than she actually should wear, frantically waving one of those old funeral parlor fans to defeat the smothering South Carolina summer heat.

Her husband, a steadfast tin soldier if ever there was one, accompanies her with smiles and patience whenever she asks him to bring her. He's always gracious and has only raised his voice at me once, during a visit when I foolishly tried to convince Toni not to use the emergency department for her ridiculous complaints. I was young and stupid. Now I don't fight it. I think of her as one of those family members one doesn't mention, but whom one can never escape.

I've seen her for chest pain, "high blood", anxiety, weakness, pelvic pain, magic spells that left her aphasic (nicely managed with droperidol) and I don't know what else. I've seen far more of her ample, middle aged body than I ever wanted to. I tried to admit her a time or two for chest pain, but she refused and by this time even refuses electrocardiograms. You see, we have a little dance, and we both know the steps.

Periodically, a new physician or nurse graces our facility and needs to be educated in how to handle Toni. The nurses and paramedics who make me the happiest understand that what she usually wants is a blood pressure check in triage and a few minutes to ventilate her unhappiness to their listening ear. She lives in a trailer without AC, so sometimes all she wants is to sit in our waiting room for an hour and cool off.

94

But even when she slips past a weak triage nurse, I don't mind so much anymore. And if I wanted, I could say, "Toni, we've got some really sick folks here. Can you come back in the morning?" She would gladly clip-clop away on her unfortunate, over-worked little heals. But now I realize that she's easily managed with a little hand patting and a few minutes of earnest listening. We have a relationship that is the closest thing I'll ever have to patient continuity in Emergency Medicine.

Once I've sifted through the chest pain or the numbness, the headache or the weakness, we get down to brass tacks. She'll say, "Docta Leap, I really think this all started after my husband and I got into a fuss. And you know my boy Carl, he got arrested this week and I been so upset. And it's so hot in my house, Docta Leap. I worries so much! I've got this collection of Elvis stuff, and this man says (whispering to me) it's worth a lot of money. I'm so afraid someone is gonna' steal it! But I'm good friends with all the policemen and I go down and sit and talk to them at the station. And they so nice to me!"

And so it goes. She feels better and I know she's fine. I show her my kid's pictures and she oohs, and ahhs. She hugs me and we part ways for a few weeks. Sometimes however, her worries are deeper, and revolve around her husband's thus far unconfirmed colon cancer, or the lady next door that died. A woman of faith in God, she shows me the prayer cloth she carries everywhere and tells me that that God will deliver her from the things she fears.

Once she told me that she would "plead the blood of Jesus" on all of us doctors. Not certain what to think at first, considering her seeming instability in matters of the mind and spirit, I decided that I was glad. Jesus spent a lot of time with the unstable, the sick, the poor, the possessed and the confused. If Toni wanted to pray for me, to cover my partners and I with the blood, then we were better off. Who knows what good things have happened because of her simple faith? Or what bad things haven't.

In Hebrews, in the New Testament, Christians are counseled "Do not forget to entertain strangers, for by so doing, some have entertained angels without knowing it." Out of the over 800 times we've seen Toni (admittedly no stranger), surely one of those was an angelic visitation, testing some bleary eyed, harried physician. I hope I was nice if it was me. I could sure use the credit.

Someday, Toni will come to one of us with a complaint that seems trivial and then return by ambulance in cardiac arrest. I can feel it. I dread it too. Not because I'm afraid of lawsuits, or databases, or anything else. I dread it because she's a part of who I am. She has educated me in the art of medicine as surely as my anatomy professors did in the science. And when she's gone, I'll miss her. I hope it's a long time from now. I'd like to see her reach at least 2400 visits before we discharge her for the last time.

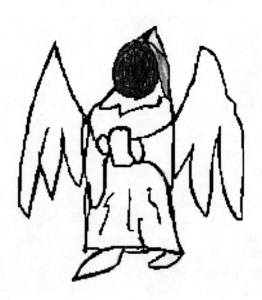

Saving Our Own Lives

An individual in our community was recently arrested after a shooting spree in his own house, his second arrest involving a weapon. No one was injured, but he was brought to the hospital for a psychiatric evaluation, then committed to a psychiatric facility. As he left, he made veiled threats about future events and it is well known that he has animosity toward the hospital and its staff. As of this writing, he is free of both commitment and incarceration, and we're scared. Why shouldn't we be? We practice in a small, rural hospital that has armed police officers for eight hours of the night, Thursday through Sunday only. Other than that, it's unarmed security with pepper spray, handcuffs and expandable batons. We don't have secure entrances and so we don't have any real effective way to prevent him from coming back and continuing his shooting spree at our facility.

Of course we can call 911. We live in a 911 society. That is, our cultural tendency is to think that whatever trouble we encounter with dangerous Homo Sapiens, the answer is a quick speed-dial to the police. The problem, as every real doctor knows, is that it only takes a second or less to fatally wound a human being, whether with a firearm, knife, blunt object or bare hands. And there are only so many laps one can run screaming around an emergency department, while being chased by a murderous lunatic until that fatal wound occurs. The police cannot magically transport themselves to our hospital to save us. They are constrained by time and space and by their day-in, day-out work of trying to keep the general community madness to a minimum. Even the tragedy at Columbine High was basically completed before law enforcement made its assault to stop the carnage.

This makes our job frightful at best. We see people all day and all night who are potentially and actually dangerous. I have learned down the years how to shake hands with and do a thorough exam on someone wearing handcuffs. But those are just the ones who have been caught. What about the others? What about the agitated, angry drunks, or the paranoid schizophrenics? What about the group of young men and women I saw late one night who, it turns out, were wanted for armed robbery in another state and considered armed and dangerous? In the face of so much danger, both malicious and psychiatric in origin, wouldn't it seem rational to protect ourselves?

I'd like us all to have police officers available all day, every day. But it usually isn't practical. I'd like us to have, at least, armed security officers. However, many hospitals are squeamish about that idea. Too often hospital security consists of well-meaning, relatively untrained retirees armed with pepper spray, handcuffs and metal batons, who generally stand back while medical personnel wrestle with violent patients. So, we're left with ourselves. Tragically, we aren't taught to defend ourselves. In fact, as a group, physicians seem to consider this an unacceptable thought. We cite our role as healers, our Hippocratic Oath, and our duty to help even the craziest and most dangerous patients. But we forget our other duties, like the ones we have to our co-workers, our rational patients, our families and most of all, our duty to ourselves. In point of fact, one of the most fundamental rights of humanity is the right of self-protection and self-preservation. But we have decided because of our great mass of psychosocial baggage that this is someone else's responsibility.

Although it's typically better when our security is left to trained professionals, there may one day be a moment when we can intervene to save our life and the lives of others. So I believe we should learn a few simple life-saving techniques. Learning is power. Physicians, nurses, paramedics and others should ask around their communities for good instructors in self-defense skills, especially the skill of identifying dangerous individuals and diffusing conflict before it starts.

There are a number of options. For the passionate, in need of a hobby and exercise, enrollment in a traditional school of martial arts that teaches Karate, Kung-Fu, Tae Kwon Do, Aikido, Ju-Jitsu (or whatever is available in the area) may be an option. It may mean taking a less traditional path like learning the Israeli system called Krav Maga, which is very street defense oriented. Or it may simply mean asking local law enforcement to give a class and frequent refreshers. The officers who live on the street know many practical ways to save their own lives, many of which can be learned easily. And they like to take care of their friends in the emergency department.

My point is not that we all become trained killers, but simply that we consider options in addition to "phone-jitsu". Sadly, we have very few. Physicians, nurses and paramedics are assaulted all the time. But the general mentality for years has been that it's just part of the job. (Try assaulting a local judge in his court to see how differently things go). We seldom press charges, administrators often don't want to make the issues public and changes usually occur only after someone is seriously injured or killed.   In the end, I think it would be better to go down struggling with my attacker than with a knife in the back while running away. Maybe I'm crazy and maybe despite 25 years of martial arts practice, I'd still be inadequate. But there's nothing wrong with being prepared. I hope none of us ever faces the situation for real. But lately, with an angry, heavily armed man running around with a vendetta toward my workplace, I guess I have to think about it.

Vulnerability of a Father

One early summer morning I saw a tragedy. It wasn't large enough for national news. It didn't concern the masses of people, who would still move quietly through their normal lives like canoes slipping through quiet water. But it was still a tragedy and sometimes, small tragedies make sharper images, more readily comprehended by observers. Unfortunately they are also more easily applied to other lives by analogy. I was an observer of this event or part of it. And although intervening in tragedy is part of my job description as a physician, this one was harder to face than most.

That morning, a young couple woke in the darkness to find that their infant son was not breathing. They called 911 and an ambulance was dispatched to their home. However, they did not wait and drove to the hospital with an urgency born of love, fear, hope and despair.

Knowing they would arrive quickly, we made preparations, opened equipment boxes, put on gloves and waited. Through the ambulance bay doors we saw a solitary car speeding towards us with lights flashing. We ran to them as a frantic, sobbing mother handed the infant, five months old, to one of our nurses. We began to work as soon he was placed on the hospital bed. A dazed father parked the car.

The infant was stiff, with the blue cast of a death that had occurred perhaps hours before. I suspected Sudden Infant Death Syndrome, SIDS. Still, we worked for a long time because it never seems like long enough when a child is involved. Every parent in the room saw their own child lying there and even as we tried to be realistic, the idea of stopping, the idea of surrendering to mortality was just too much. In the end we knew what we had to do. One of the results of years of practice, as a nurse or physician, is the ability to know death when you see it. We looked at the clock, looked at one another and stopped.

There's always a painful silence when a resuscitation ends. Medical television shows can't reproduce it. The quiet rhythm of chest compressions, reflected in beeps on the heart monitor, ceases. The sound of artificial breathing is gone. The tearing open of medications, the flow of orders and confirmations, the nervousness in the voices of the staff, all suddenly quiet. The monitor silently draws a flat, green, electric line, then prints a strip of paper with a flat line for the record. It is switched off without ceremony, without any requiem to mark the end.

Whether the deceased was child or adult, I usually stand a slight distance away from their body and look at them from head to toe. I try to take them in, to log them in my memory. Not out of morbid fascination, but to somehow preserve a bit of them, or imagine them alive, or to honor their humanity in the solitude of my mind, like some brief memorial service. Looking at this child, I saw that he was beautiful. He was fair and came to us dressed only in a diaper. He was perfect in form. As a father of three young sons, I remembered this age. Five months is an age of rolling, laughing and recognition. It is an age of bonding, rocking and early play. It is an age in which you still marvel at the indescribable softness of infant skin, the sweet smell of warm infant breath as a child lies on your chest asleep. I saw my children before me, and prayed quietly that they were safe at home, even as I had prayed that this child would live and that his parents' hearts would survive, as he had not.

I managed to suppress the internal analogies to my own sons. I accepted the inevitable internal review. The "what else could I have done" that always comes. I trained for all of this. Still, the worst part was the last. The walk down the hall to parents who sat waiting for news. As I stepped into the conference room with one of the nurses, I saw the mother, tear streaked, rocking silently back and forth in her chair. The father, still stunned, on the phone with family. I sat down and explained what had happened. They expected it, I think. They wept openly, but I think they knew when they picked him up, cold in a warm bed, that he was gone from them. My heart broke too.

Then a stunning thing happened. I had called the child by the wrong name, which had somehow been given to the clerk at the desk. The father corrected me and took my breath away. His name means, "The Lord is my God," in Hebrew. It is also the name of my 15-month-old son.

I was shaken. I told them how sorry I was. In eleven years of practice I haven't yet learned to cry with families, but I was close that day. I needed desperately to leave the room. I finished the shift as the stream of other family members came and went to the room where their child lay.

Finally, I went home to my wife and boys. As I walked in the door they mobbed me as only little boys can. My son was laughing and running with his brothers, still in pajamas from the night. I picked him up and held him close to me. He gave me an obligatory snuggle, squirmed away and was off for more wrestling and squealing. But while I held him I marveled and rejoiced in his life. And mourned for the other child and his parents.

Fatherhood is unbelievable. It is a daily exercise in joy. It is loving, nurturing, teaching, playing, laughing, crying, punishing and rewarding. It is so many things. And as modern fathers we have learned things our fathers, and theirs, never knew about the joy of involvement in our children's lives. But one of the things we seldom hear about is the curse of fatherhood, which is vulnerability.

I sometimes think that our ancestors, recent and distant, were smarter than we think. We too often condemn them retroactively for their absence in child rearing. But perhaps it was a habit developed long ago, by men who knew too well the pain of loss, when children's deaths were all too common. They knew that their wives would be crushed by loss, but maybe felt that distance would protect them from pain in a time when men's emotions were things they understood little and articulated even less. And when stoic strength was the way men coped with their pain.

I suspect that they knew well that once we have loved fully, once we have surrendered entirely to a consuming passion for our children, we are somehow hostages. Whatever happens to them will affect us forever and in tragedy bring us closer to destruction than anything ever could have before. I don't like this part of fatherhood, which looms over me every day of my life.

I was so affected by my vulnerability that day that I could not tell my wife the whole story. I skirted the issue, mentioned a SIDS death in our morning debrief over breakfast and went on. I wanted to tell her what I had felt. But in my personal neurosis, feared that to mention it would somehow call down danger on my child. This is one of the irrational thoughts stored in the cabinet of fear that I keep as a parent. I try to keep it shut, but sometimes events unlock it and the door swings wide as horrible daydreams and nightmares combine to fill me with paralyzing anxiety about my children's lives.

Fatherhood is an expensive venture. It costs us far more than money. It costs us our time, our youth, our energy and our freedom. But the most burdensome part, for me, is the price of vulnerability. And as I looked into the eyes of that child's father and mother, I saw that they had paid the ultimate price of love, far higher than I, as abstract vulnerability became horrible reality. I prayed all that day for them. And I prayed that I would never fully understand their pain.

Making a House Call

Not too long ago I made a house call. As a physician accustomed to working in the emergency department of a hospital, this was quite a change of pace. But it involved friends and their sick child and it was a joy. We had spoken on the phone and I had some concerns about their infant, who had developed a high fever. When I went to their home I took only my stethoscope and my experience as a physician and parent of four.

When I walked through the door on Friday evening there were candles burning as dinner was prepared. There were no florescent lights. There was none of the chaos of a waiting room. No ambulances idled outside. No bloody, angry drunk screamed profanities. No one stood by the exam room door, arms crossed in annoyance with waiting. It was a quiet place to be; and the child, on his worried mother's hip, was quiet as well. He was in a place where he felt safe and was thus able to tolerate my poking and prodding.

I examined him and decided that he was not seriously ill. Because his mother had described him as lethargic when we spoke, I had been concerned that he might have meningitis. This was not actually the case. His parents and I were obviously relieved.

After he was dosed with ibuprofen and put to bed, I chatted a while with his mom and dad, then left for home. As I drove home I realized that, although the family had thanked me, it was I who owed them thanks. I owed them thanks for helping me to realize the essence of what I do and for letting me enjoy it in such a peaceful setting.

What was it that made this so different from my day-to-day practice? I asked myself this question and realized that there were many answers. For one thing it was voluntary. This is very important. Medicine today is so much under the control of private and government regulatory agencies that practice always seems compulsory. Of course, I do my job by choice. But federal law says that I must see everyone who comes through the door, without any promise of payment. For most patients, this is fine. But there are some that I wish I had the option to refuse, because they repeatedly abuse a system designed to protect them. Furthermore, this visit did not involve any sort of entitlement. The child's parents did not say to me "I have a right to your care! You owe me your expertise!" My services still had value. Entitlement to health care, or anything, cheapens it in the end and opens the door to its abuse.

Further, it did not involve any paperwork. Modern charting is a nightmare. It must be done correctly for legal reasons, in case a patient encounter ends up in court. It must be done correctly for billing reasons, because (especially with Medicare) if a chart is not dictated or written according to a meticulous and complex formula, then appropriate payment is denied. My house call was free and I would have been insulted by any offer of compensation. But the labyrinthine regulations imposed by the government have made reimbursement in my normal practice very difficult. Worse, incorrect billing, even if it involves an honest mistake, is now viewed as fraudulent. Physicians can be investigated by the government for charging too much or too little. Likewise, paperwork must be done properly to avoid other federal legal entanglements. A simple transfer form filled out incorrectly can result in tens of thousands of dollars in federal fines and loss of Medicare participation. To the federal government, there are no accidents, only criminal acts.

I'm not whining, I'm lamenting. I'm lamenting the passing of an era when being a physician was not only a privilege, but a pleasure. Some people believe that the only answers to medicine's problems involve the increasing intervention of government and industry to regulate the activity of physicians. This is tragic. Because it robs physicians of the sustaining professional virtues of honor, compassion and duty to humanity, and replaces them with legalistic guidelines devised by middle management and civil functionaries; persons who have never experienced the joys and sorrows of the wonderful profession they seek to regulate.

I suppose it is no wonder house-calls are rare. The nostalgia they invoke may just be too painful to bear.

It's Better Incognito

Sitting in Ruby Tuesday's Restaurant with my family, a very pleasant, well spoken lady looked across from a nearby booth and said, "Don't I know you from somewhere?" My wife and I held our breath for a second. As an emergency physician, one never knows what the next line will be. My encounters with patients and their families are limited. I seldom get much follow-up on outcomes of my patients when they leave the hospital. My mind raced: "You sent my father home the night before he died" Argh. "I developed a huge scar on my face after you sutured my cut!" Ugh. "I had a horrible reaction to the medicine you gave me. You'll be hearing from my attorney." Ouch.

Fortunately, that hasn't happened. I mean, I know people have bad outcomes. It's inevitable in medicine, just like a car keeps making that weird noise even after the mechanic fixes it. Nevertheless, patients say very gracious things to me in public. Or, they don't recognize me, which is just as well. Like many who work with the public, anonymity is a trait I have cultivated. I don't wear the "doctor uniform" in public. No stethoscope, no pager, no pen or tie with a caduceus on it. I almost never introduce myself as doctor. It works well.

But this lady had me. So I volunteered, "Have you been to the ER lately?" "That's it! I was there this weekend with a student from (Unnamed) University! You were so nice!" I smiled. This was going to be an easy one. Lunch would go on undisturbed except for my little nephew walking out of the bathroom naked.

She went on. "But you know, that little doctor we saw, he just wasn't, well, we were just disappointed. I mean, people who come to the ER are a little weird, I know that, but he just wasn't nice. He tapped on that girl's forehead and she pushed him away and he tapped again and she slapped his hand off. And he said, 'I'm just trying to do my job'. But that nurse made up for it. She was so nice. And you were so nice! Thank you!"

The sound of my deflating ego was audible. I smiled and shook my head in understanding. Tempted to say that I was the doctor, I realized she would have been mortified. Jan and I had to contain our laughter. I'm not sure who she thought I was. Registration clerk?

Housekeeping? Security? Strange little man walking from room to room shaking hands?

It was obvious that I had not met her expectations, or those of the patient. I suppose it's good for me to get knocked down now and then. I pride myself on being "Mister nice-guy". My co-workers would actually back me up on this. I try hard to take everyone seriously, or at least act like it. I attempt to speak in quiet-tones, and to sit and listen as long as I have time. I like for people to feel that I have given them quality care. But this time, I guess I dropped the ball.

What actually happened? The young lady had a high fever and probably felt terrible. I was tapping on her apparently infected sinuses and I'm sure it hurt. It was busy. I must have been abrupt. I'm glad that the nice lady in the restaurant pointed out my behavior. We all need course corrections in life's journey now and then.

However, her critique gave me an idea. I've decided that I need to change the way I answer that question, "don't I know you?" Jan and I discussed a whole list of possible answers. She has some good ideas, that wife of mine. After all, she's the one who when her 9 month pregnant abdomen was stroked by a stranger at the local Mall, said "I'm not pregnant, I'm just fat!"

So here are the winners: "You might know me. My name is Bruno. I'm an exotic dancer." "Do we have the same parole officer?" "Is my picture still on that milk carton?" And last but not least, "That was probably my twin brother. Is he still pretending to be a doctor?"

Prescription for Hypocrisy

Among the many issues tossed about in medical politics, Medicare occupies a prominent place. What to do to save it? How to extend its coverage? Whether or not to provide prescription drug coverage? Physicians are "in the belly of the beast" on this one. Few of us can afford to opt out of Medicare, so we are faced with an increasingly complex maze of regulations regarding utilization and reimbursement, many of which, if poorly understood (much less blatantly ignored) can result in fines and imprisonment. Things sure have changed.

But, in spite of it all, in the face of a growing retiree population, it's obvious that Medicare is important and will continue to be. Therefore, I submit that all of the rules and laws, burdensome and illogical, ridiculous, punitive and costly though they may be, are necessary. We should not try to resist. We should submit, for the common good. Because even if we are innocent of any wrongdoing, even if we have never committed either error or fraud, even if we never will, someone will; and sometimes collective punishment is the only way to achieve the end desired for the good of society as a whole. And indeed, if the government says that I have committed a crime, who am I to say otherwise? We must accept, as we move towards a more profound and encompassing statism, that our elected and appointed officials have only our best interest in mind and would never act on incomplete or poorly formulated information. I am innocent. But for the good of all, punish me if needed and I will be happy to serve the state.

Now, if you've read this far without tearing out the page, please continue. All that claptrap I just recited is fabricated. (Although I think I might try to memorize it for the time when I'm sent to the new order medical re-education camp). I made it up to make a point. The first paragraph is true. Medicine is full of political concerns. But the one I want to address is not Medicare. It's gun control.

Emergency physicians, using a public health/injury control model, have placed themselves at the forefront of the debate on gun control. This is a topic of visceral importance to many Americans. The emergency medicine establishment has, as a rule, dismissed gun advocates as lunatics, gun-nuts, rednecks and cretins and has used statistical data to try to formulate policy affecting millions, all the while blatantly ignoring the will and freedoms of those who own, use and enjoy firearms in America.

Now, I went on and on in that second paragraph about accepting collective punishment, because that is what American gun owners are being asked to do. Some 80,000,000 of us, with an estimated 250,000,000 firearms, are being told that we should subject ourselves to ever more draconian and invasive gun control legislation, even though we have never committed a crime, even though we have never had an accident. Considering that gun crimes and accidents are at their lowest point in years, calls for aggressive restrictions are simply more evidence that the agenda is driven by social engineering far more than it is driven by public health concerns.

Gun control has a unique position in America today. If it is imposed in a municipality or state and crime drops, it is hailed as the answer and calls for more gun control echo through the media, academia and government. However, if it fails and crime climbs or stays the same, the call is for tighter gun control. This "positively reinforcing feedback loop" never ends. It only gets bigger and more powerful. And it is obvious from the views of members of, again; media, government, academia and medicine, that the goal is ultimately nothing short of (in order of their progression) licensing of all gun owners, total registration of all firearms, storage laws, needs-based licensing (not to include self defense) and ultimately, though it is seldom mentioned yet, confiscation. For almost all registration schemes have the potential to end in confiscation. The much praised registration systems of England and Australia resulted in the horrific confiscation of lawfully registered shotguns, rifles and handguns (even .22 caliber target arms) from lawful owners, for no other reason than philosophical differences between power elite and gun owners. Their crime rates were already minuscule so what was the point?

And what has happened now that our enlightened friends in England surrendered their lawful arms? Violent crime has increased dramatically. As an example, I read once that Manchester, England had been referred to as "Gunchester", because so many young criminals have access to black market firearms, stolen from collections and smuggled from Eastern Europe. Now it may be true that one would need to study this carefully to establish causality. This is, after all, the rallying cry of gun control advocates. But my point, as a non-statistician, is simply this. Even if there were no direct effect and no causality, crime still went up and good citizens were debarred the ownership and simple pleasure of their lawful arms. Similar effects have been experienced in Australia, a country with a long history of lawful firearms ownership. Sixty percent of Australian firearms were outlawed in 1997. Then, violent crime increased dramatically. According to an article by Miguel A. Faria, Jr., MD in Medical Sentinel, the homicide rate in the State of Victoria, Australia, rose 300% the year after harsh gun control measures were instituted. Similar increases have been experienced across the country.

And yet, the goal of gun control in America is clearly that of bans and confiscation based on the much venerated "European model". And it will progress with great speed unless gun owners stand against it. I know that many physicians are avid gun owners. I am and have known physicians who owned many firearms, some simple double barreled shotguns for bird hunting, some fully automatic submachine guns legally owned with proper federal paperwork. Never have I known any of them to 1) commit a crime, or 2) have an accident. Physician gun owners must stand up to those in our profession who would use their medical badge to bully lawful citizens into surrendering a freedom that has been passed down since the founding of the land. You see, I don't really care what they do anywhere else. I don't live there. America is unique in the history of the world and part of that unique quality is that government is counterbalanced by an armed populace.

This is far more than an issue of studies and statistics, for there are also convincing statistics that support gun ownership as a deterrent to crime. I'm not going to go there, except to say that wherever concealed carry laws have been instituted, one thing is certain. Those who hold permits do not commit crimes. The data does not need statistical manipulation. It is straightforward. States with permits for concealed carry revoke those permits for crimes committed, and it simply isn't happening. Those states which allow such permits (31 so far) have not noted any trend toward violence among those who lawfully own and carry. Further, areas with high rates of gun ownership and concealed carry enjoy decreasing violent crime.

I wonder how many physicians who enjoy a bottle of fine wine or beer with dinner, or who make or collect wine or beer, consider themselves as contributing to drunken driving and alcohol related violent behavior. Maybe, as a good faith effort, they should subject themselves to a "one beer a week" rule. Or perhaps to a "license to purchase" alcohol that shows that they have never been convicted of driving under the influence. (It would be a simple matter. A short class on the dangers of alcohol, an application with fingerprints and photos, a background check and a fee. After such licensing, no one would drink and drive, because they couldn't obtain alcohol, right?). Doubtless many would cry that their civil rights were infringed, or would say, "I never drink and drive! This isn't my fault!" My point exactly. For physicians to suggest that the government intervene in private life more than it already does is surely a prescription for hypocrisy.

You see, this is an issue of ideology. And though some consider themselves such scientific purists that ideology is irrelevant to their social agenda and sneer at persons like myself for our use of such intangibles as "freedom", "liberty" and "security", I believe that ideology is relevant. And I believe that when we, as physicians, begin to treat the public as if they are simple children to be hemmed in and protected against their own will, the will of 80,000,000 persons, we do them a far greater disservice than we imagine. We should be the guardians of individual autonomy. Instead, we become lap dogs of big government and contribute to the advancing tyranny of statism; willing foot soldiers in an army of paternalistic oppression, masquerading as public health.

As I sit in my back yard in rural South Carolina and fire my rifle, I am stricken by the ignorance of so many physicians. Many of them would doubtless say that I risk my family's life simply by having any firearm. They don't care that my grandmother defended her life with a firearm when she was in her 70's. They don't care that no one in my family has ever had an accidental injury or death from a firearm (or committed a crime with one) for as far back as I know. They do not,

111

nor will they ever understand, that like any tool, it is to be treated with respect, no less than a circular saw. And worse, they will never understand the joy of the feel of my firearm in my hands, the crack of the bullet discharging, the hole in the target, or the smell of powder. This is a heritage passed down for hundreds of years. It should not be surrendered lightly, no matter what our well-meaning colleagues may say, nor how condescending their arguments.

Getting Stoned (in the Kidney)

Every now and then it's a good thing for a doctor to be a patient. I always like to be able to tell patients that I understand their illness. I always liked it, that is, until that fateful day when I had my kidney stone.

It was a normal Monday morning, as I attempted to conduct family business on a day off. My wife, then 22 weeks pregnant with our third (though not our final) child, was riding herd on the two yard-apes, as well as another, our nephew. I was sitting in my chair, phone in hand when I felt the first twinge. Twisting, I dismissed it as a pulled muscle. Twinge again. I shifted my seat and attempted to make a call. Then there were no more twinges; there was just agony. I began to pant and as the shooting, hot-iron pain ran from my back to my abdomen my highly educated, well trained analytical mind said those two words I long dreaded and had so hoped to avoid, "Drugs please!"

That it was a kidney stone was clear to me as I walked, bent double, to my wife. She has accompanied me in one way or another through my entire education and probably knows about as much medicine as I do. She looked at me and said, calmly, "do I need to take you to the hospital?" "Yes please", I said with a weak, grateful smile.

So, we dressed the children, loaded them in the car and headed down the road. I squeezed her hand and panted as she apologized for not paying much attention in Lamaze class. She was a wonderful coach actually and the analogy is not lost, since women who have had children and kidney stones say that they were equivalent, some giving the stone the blue ribbon prize for pain.

The 10-minute drive to Oconee Memorial Hospital seemed a bit longer, by about a million years, as waves of spasm passed down my ureter. She let me out and drove the children around since it was near nap-time. I walked into the ER, where my colleagues were busily doing their jobs. Apparently I was pale as a sheet because one of our nurses, who is also a good friend, stepped back and said "Don't throw up on me! What's wrong with you?" This sort of Florence Nightingale compassion is very comforting in the face of pain. When I explained my dilemma, she laughed and started my IV. (We have long wagered who would have gallstones first and this was almost as good in her book).

My partner ordered the sweet nectar Demerol, mixed with Phenergan for nausea and the long dream began. I have been told that I wouldn't shut up while the lights were on, but that when they were out and everyone left the room, I drifted off quite nicely. Next, another dear friend and nurse of extraordinary compassion cared for me. I have always been impressed by our nurses, but am more so having personally relied on their kindness and ability.

More medicine was administered and I left for Xray to look for the location and condition of the stone. Someone asked me "were they nice to you in X-ray?" They could have beaten me with ball bats, taken my wallet and dressed me in drag. I never would have cared. Sleeping on an X-ray table was never so sweet. No wonder people ask me for Demerol so often!

When all was said and done and I was back in the emergency department, my partner and my good friend the radiologist stood by me. The radiologist said that I had one stone about to pass and "two or three more on the launching pad". That seemed so horrible in my drugged state that I will never forget it. What launching pad? Has the countdown started?

That evening, back home and pain free, I began to reflect. What did I learn? Being in severe pain is always bad. Narcotics are magic. Good doctors and nurses are gifts directly from God himself. And the availability of emergency care in America, 24 hours a day, seven days a week, makes all the complaints about health care in the US seem weak and paltry.

And I learned that when anyone comes to me with a kidney stone, a genuine, honest to goodness kidney stone, they should get whatever they need. Because brother, it really hurts. And that ain't no lie.

Did You Hear the One About the Lawyer?

The graduation ceremony of the University of Georgia School of Law, that I attended this past spring, was a study in contrasts. As a physician, I could recall such days myself; days of fulfillment, of dreams realized. Before me, on the bright green grass of a common, under shady Southern Oaks by the school itself, freshly educated law students lined up to accept their diplomas. After years of work, these idealistic young men and women were about to sally forth into society to right wrongs, stamp out oppression and eagerly document billable hours. Touching as it was, I felt a little like I had stumbled onto a scene of unspeakable evil. I had discovered the spawning ground of the legions of darkness.

But I wasn't there as a spy for the world of medicine. I was there to watch my wife's sister graduate. And I simply couldn't imagine her as a "minion of evil." I've seen her smiling, enthusiastic face too many times. I've known her since she was a child, and have watched her mind, faith and ethics develop to ever higher levels. Drat, she's a nice lawyer.

The truth is, I've met many nice lawyers. Not only Julie, my wife Jan's sister, but Angela, my best friend from high school. And Brad and Scott, with whom we have supper club with once a month. Like us, lawyers are mostly men and women who want to make a living and care for their families. Most of them mean what they say about truth and justice, to the extent that we physicians always see ourselves as "healers". I suppose that lawyers, like physicians, learn over the years how to fuse ideals and reality into a functioning whole. Just as seasoned physicians don't run screaming into exam rooms when someone says "chest pain", attorneys don't drop everything and race to court just because someone says "no fair!" or "Doctor off the port bow, battle stations!" Reality does its work on all of us.

And here's another reality. Physicians and attorneys help to keep the rest of society functioning. It's easy to see our professions as ends in themselves, but they aren't. I have described physicians, myself included, as "mechanics for humans". We train and practice to help humans continue working, playing and loving for as long as they can.

So it is with our fellow professionals in law. They serve society so that persons can live within the laws of the land with as little trouble as possible. It is their job to keep the law reasonable and save us from the oppression of unjust rulers. It is their job to protect us from the misuse of evil persons and organizations that would rob us of life, freedom or property. They take the abstract concept of justice and allow real people access to its benefits, so that they can be free of the distractions of duels, revenge or any of the other means that societies have used to remedy wrongs in less enlightened ages. Attorneys serve a law that is not an end, but a means.

As we move through our careers it's easy to deride other professions. Sometimes it's a fun joke, like a "doctor/lawyer" basketball game. Other times it's a stone-wall preventing what could be a healthy interaction. And it happens more easily when traditional enemies use insulting names, rather than attach real faces to titles.

I can more readily call a lawyer a "lousy ambulance chaser" when I don't know the sound of his laughter, the name of his wife or the faces of his children. Likewise, a physician makes a more handy target for a lawsuit when viewed as little more than a "rich doctor", without the knowledge that he sometimes gives away free care, misses his wife and children when he works and isn't so rich after all.

I'll probably keep telling lawyer jokes, at least good ones. My lawyer friends will still tell doctor jokes. But I wish that across the country, both professions could learn to recognize their relative importance, or lack thereof, to the forward motion of the country. After all, it's just a matter of perspective.

The Real Power of Medicine

Medicine is facing enormous changes. Every day new regulations pass, new laws are instituted, new markets consumed by powerful managed care organizations. As this occurs physicians sometimes feel overwhelmed. We are, by our very nature, poor administrators and politicians (although exceptions fortunately exist). We spend years becoming adept at the science of medicine, but seldom become familiar with the management of medicine until it is too late. Some, disgusted with the entire effort, simply quit. They feel that the problems of finance and litigation make the practice of medicine an unworthy pursuit. Many of us at times feel completely out of control of our destinies, as decisions are continually taken away and we become so many puppets in the great show.

But there is a way. There is an avenue we can travel which will forever subvert the intense pressures of market and law and usurp the hold of middle managers in health care. We can return to our calling and begin again to love our profession and our patients.

No matter how many MBA's stand between us and the patient; no matter how many attorneys threaten us with financial devastation and career ending lawsuits, we are still the ones who touch the dying. We are still the ones who alleviate the pain of the sick and injured, who comfort the minds of worry stricken parents. For ages we have been integral to human existence. Whether as tribal shaman or as highly trained sub-specialists, we have existed to bring comfort, hope and occasionally healing. We are in a position of great nobility.

Although emergency care is frequently frustrating, it is also full of reminders of why the medical profession in general is so grand. Sometimes patients or their families look at me and say, "I was just scared"; then I realize that even the function of saying "nothing is wrong" is a great opportunity. Fear is a powerful emotion and fear of illness or injury is one of the most potent. When we can lift the weight of fear and replace it with hope, we reach deep into the souls of our brothers and sisters.

There are also those times when physicians actually can heal. The patient with a heart attack who lives on to have a full life, the cancer victim who overcomes, the fracture repaired, the simple toothache anesthetized, the earache soothed; these are moments of glory, when we can combine knowledge with art, science with love and rise to the high place to which we originally aspired as idealistic students.

But there are also those times when pain wins in spite of our efforts, when death breaches the weak defenses of our primitive skills and knowledge. In those moments of weeping or suffering, when loss is monumental and defeat looms before the helpless, we can offer our hand, our genuine grief, our gentility. It is then that we can most emulate the Great Physician and be an ally in the struggle eternal. Then we can show patients that we truly care more for them than we do for money or status.

No one in government, no one in the insurance industry has any access to that power. It lies within our minds and souls, it is mirrored in our eyes and it is expressed in our touch. If we think that we no longer have the place in society we once had, we are wrong. We sometimes just forget why we had it in the first place.

What we have forgotten is that humans revere greatness, knowledge and power but hold highest those whose greatness stems from service. Mighty Julius Caesar has gone to dust and his words are most often known only to Latin students; who as I did, mostly forget them. The words of Christ, however, have guided much of mankind for two millennia, showing no signs of decay. He led no legions, won no battles and submitted to a criminal's execution. But His love, expressed so humbly, made him beloved in the hearts of everyone who knew him or has known him since.

If we physicians hope to secure our place in the hearts of humankind, we need only remember what an incredible honor and privilege it is to dress the wounds of mankind. Seen through this lens, the modern problems of the profession seem minute and easily overcome.

Everyone is Fighting a Great Battle

Lying on the exam table was a young woman in her mid to late thirties. She was a little anxious. Her chart indicated that she had back pain, neck pain, headache, chest pain and insomnia. I took a deep breath, rolled my eyes and began to take a history. I tried my best to tease out what things might be serious and what not. No injuries, no weakness, no shortness of breath, no history of heart disease, no thunderclap headaches, no, no, no. Her exam was almost as unremarkable. Until we went a little further.

As her history continued and she opened up, I learned that she was working third shift at a local factory, raising three small children and caring for a husband on dialysis, awaiting a kidney transplant. No wonder she had insomnia! She didn't have time to sleep.

It would have been very easy for me, once serious problems were ruled out, to brusquely explain that the emergency department was not the place for her multiple complaints. That she should see a primary care physician. That I had nothing to offer her. Some nights, with other patients, I have doubtless done this.

Fortunately I didn't say that to her, although I don't recall many details of our visit. I may have been busy, or may not. Her name escapes me. I may have given her some hydroxyzine for sleep, or a referral to mental health, or a suggestion that she turn to a church for some assistance. But it's irrelevant.

I know that I let her vent and told her that many of her symptoms were probably related to stress and fatigue. I think she needed that. The truth can be liberating and too often we fail to give it to patients. We dance around, inventing diagnoses and ignoring the obvious, when they look to us for honest answers. Honest answers can be uncomfortable, but are also one of the greatest prescriptions we can give. Even though her problems remained (even though I couldn't write a "please excuse from life" note), I think that she went away a little reassured. Maybe all she needed to hear was that she wasn't dying.

However, I'm not writing about honesty, or about meeting the cornucopia of psycho-social needs that present to us every day in busy emergency departments. We aren't psychologists, pastors, counselors, or rabbis, though occasionally we're forced to act like them. We're physicians trained to intervene in life and limb threatening medical emergencies. The demands of modern emergency care are so great that it is an unusual day when we can sit and delve deeply into a patient's life, beyond "are you hearing voices or thinking of killing yourself?"

Of course, we are constantly reminded that in addition to providing state of the art medical care, attempting to know the drug interactions between the dozens of bottles of prescriptions our patients take, reducing our rate of errors, avoiding litigation, billing Medicare correctly and participating in political advocacy, we should also take a little time to counsel our patients/ "customers" about domestic violence, immunizations, alcohol abuse and other issues. Small wonder that patients' hidden agendas and subtexts slip past us; we simply can't do it all.

But there's one thing we can do and that's what I'm writing about. We can treat everyone with kindness. This is harder to quantify; it isn't easily studied in double-blind, placebo controlled, cross-over studies. It can't be readily evaluated on satisfaction surveys. It doesn't lend itself to quality assurance meetings. Administrators aren't comfortable with sending out a memo saying, "Let's all be a little kinder". Furthermore, kindness is difficult. It can require a major effort of the soul to step out of the single-minded vision of our own schedule, or our own anger and slow down long enough to speak gently, or touch a child with a reassuring hand.

But that's the beauty of it. Kindness, an unquantifiable quantity, helps us to care for our fellow humans with compassion as well as competence and the combination is powerful. Kindness is voluntary, so those physicians who opt for it will, in the end, rise up above their peers. But not necessarily in ways that lead to position or profit, which too often favor cruelty or cold efficiency. They will rise in ways imperceptible to the concrete markers of professional life. They will rise up in the hearts of the patients they care for and (I believe) in the estimation of their Creator, whose children they are charged with healing and helping. My college physics professor, Dr. Bellis, put it perfectly when he said, "Ah, but the reward for virtue is not in this life".

Early last year I came across a quotation from another very wise man. His name was Philo of Alexandria, and he was a renowned Jewish scholar who lived at the beginning of the first millennium. He said, "Be kind, for everyone you meet is fighting a great battle". He knew something about battles. In the year 40 CE he was sent to the Roman Emperor Caligula, whose disposition was far worse than anyone from HCFA, to plead the case of Jews mistreated by Gentiles. He lived in a time when conquest and cruelty were the norm. Doubtless he experienced a fair amount himself in the 70 years he lived. Still, he came to the conclusion that everyone's life is difficult and that one of the best ways to treat people well is to remember that we do not always know what lies beneath the surface, behind their public face.

Although it is often very, very hard, I've tried to remember these sage words that came to me down 2000 years. Some nights, with some people, it's as if Philo himself had said those words for me, to help me have perspective. Because I sure can complain and in my complaining, too often believe that my life is dramatically more difficult than the lives of my patients. But at the end of the day, I get in my car, drive to my home and see my family. That alone separates me from untold numbers of persons whose lives are total disarray and daily tragedy. Furthermore, although I see a lot of patients for free, I'll still receive a good paycheck for the month and have money in retirement, insurance for my family's illnesses and a little extra for luxuries like vacations.

I fight my battles, but they're mostly skirmishes with inconvenience. My job puts me in touch with persons whose battles are, without question, to the death. They battle with the world and more often with themselves. The one thing I can do is show a little kindness, whether or not I make them better. In the end it will help them and elevate me. And if I can finish a shift having accomplished those two goals, my patients and I will all have profited.

Coping with My Fear of the Night

I work full time nights. There is a method to my madness. By doing this, I work less shifts and have more days off each month to spend with my wife our four children. Nights in the emergency department are seldom as slow as I'd like. They usually challenge my skill and my patience. But even more, they challenge my faith. Because over the years, I seem to have developed a growing sense of vague anxiety. It isn't debilitating. And maybe it is just fatherhood. But every night when I leave for work, I fear. And, as I fear I allow doubt to creep into my thoughts and erode my faith like a slow growing cancer.

I suppose the practice of medicine in modern times is enough to engender anxiety. Although I do not work at an urban trauma center, I trained at one. Furthermore, I see enough terrible, frightening things to cause anyone to fear. And what I do not see, I imagine. Even a partial list would be exhaustive, but among the things that I fear most are violence or accidents involving my family and medical errors or failures on my part that might cost someone their life. However, over the past year I have discovered a strategy. It came from two sources of inspiration.

First, one day as I was thinking about how many of my patients are frustrating or difficult, I seemed to hear God speak to me. He said, ever so quietly, "You take care of my children and I'll take care of yours". I think he meant that while all of the patients I see are his sons and daughters, some of them, perhaps the most frustrating ones, are his problem children. They are his prodigals. And for some, my partners and I are the only persons who give them medical care. Some of them are trapped by substance abuse, some by domestic violence, others by poverty or ignorance. But whatever the problem, he still loves them. And when they are sick or injured, he wants them cared for not just with competence, but with compassion. He seemed to be explaining an arrangement, as it were. Just as I want God to give mercy to my wife and sons and daughter (and myself), he wants me to give mercy to these, his special children. In the midst of caring for them, this reality gives me pause, and helps me to remember that their father is the king.

Second, I began to see that prayer is the antidote to fear and nourishment for faith. But the hectic pace of raising three young sons combined, with a full time practice, often makes prolonged periods of prayer and reflection very difficult. However I came to realize, by reading Richard Foster's book "Prayer", that these things are possible if we accept that they may look a little different, or happen in unique ways that fit our lifestyles. Sometimes they can only come twice a week, sometimes several times, but in shorter bursts. With this in mind, I developed the habit of praying in my car before leaving for work each night. Sitting in the dark, I pray with two basic intentions. First, I pray for the safety and peace of my family throughout the night. I think that the Psalmist understood this well, when he said, in Psalm 91: 5-6 "You will not fear the terror of night...nor the pestilence that stalks in the darkness...". I ask for him to watch over each of them as I list them by name. Next, I pray for the patients that I will see in the coming hours. I ask that God keep them from critical illness or injury. But, whatever their problem, I ask him to guide me and make me capable and kind as I try to meet their needs.

Now when I leave for work, I have this time of comfort. It gives me peace. It eases my anxiety on virtually every level, personal and professional. I know I do not deserve any special protection from Him. But I ask for it anyway. And because he is my father, I trust him. As a father, I know that just the chance to talk puts my little ones' fears away. I suppose it should be no surprise that the same is true for me.

So, I'm coming to grips with my anxiety. It was important first to embrace and accept it. As physicians, we have been too often educated in an environment that denied our own fear, branding it weakness. But every great man and woman of the Bible knew fear, even Jesus himself. But they were not possessed by it. So, I've learned to practice and live, in the presence of my fears, but without staring too long at them. They are, after all, mostly shadows of much smaller things. And God can handle them all.

What do you call an Emergency Physician?

Emergentologist?   A bit stuffy, frankly

How about the following, based on the realities of the job?

Alcohologist (I don't drink alcohol, just beer)

Analgesiologist (Ain't you go no pain pills?)

Dispositionist (At 2 AM, I can disposition anything)

Regulatologist (HIPPA, EMTALA, JCAHO, etc.)

Altercationist (Some dudes beat me up)

Consultationist (I don't know what it is, but I know someone who might!)

Anxiatrist (My nerves is all tore up)

Paresthesiologist (I'm tingling doc!)

Narcotologist (Only thing that works for me is Vicodin!)

Deceptionist (I swear, I don't know how that ventilator ended up in my car!)

Geriatro-behaviorologist (Grandma ain't acting right)

Mortologist (Would you mind pronouncing someone dead for me?)

What else do you call an emergency department?

Work avoidance department (Before I go, can I get a work excuse?)

College Student Post-Party observation department (Yes, Tiffany is pretty drunk, but she'll be fine!)

Pre-Incarceration evaluation center (Son, you can go to jail, or to the ER. What do you want to do?)

Pre-litigation processing center (My lawyer said to get some x-rays)

Narcotic Dealer re-supply depot (I swear, this groundhog snatched my pill bottle!)

The Epiphany Place (I'll tell you one thing, I ain't gonna kiss no more rattlesnakes!)

The Gifts of the Dead

Sometimes, when the emergency room is slow, a physician on staff will call me in the middle of the night and ask a favor. "Hey Ed, Mrs. L. died up on fourth floor. Do you have time to pronounce her for me?" I really don't mind. It's a courtesy that I can always refuse, but seldom do unless I'm very busy. But I've always found it odd, not due to the dead, but the living. I am secretly delighted when the family has already gone home. After all, they know the score from the nurses, I just make it official. Besides, I never know what to say. "Hello strangers! I'm here to make sure grandma is actually, not partly, dead. So let me interrupt your grief to listen to her chest, roll back her eyelids, and slip my hand under the covers to pinch her. It will only take a second. Smoke 'em if you got 'em!" It's awkward, to be the unknown doctor in such circumstances. But over time I've learned how to speak to these family members; how to shake their hands and touch them with some sincerity. It's an outgrowth of the part of emergency medicine that involves walking up to total strangers to tell them that a loved one has died, abruptly, horribly, then walking away never to see them again. It's blitzkrieg intimacy.

But when the family isn't there, I find myself stepping back and looking for a few moments at the person who has passed. Often, it's only the two of us in the room. I figure I won't see them again until the Great Judgment, so we'll take a moment or two together. After all, my name will be on their records from then on and usually I am with them in the darkness of late night or early morning. The fee I charge for this last doctor's visit is a farthing of reflection, a few gold coins of wisdom from the western isles.

And so I do the dance, evaluating a man or woman who I know is already gone. Now, I'm sure that honest mistakes have been made about death. You know, "Local man wakes up in morgue". But really, death is a thing that becomes so evident when one has seen it enough. To the uninitiated, near death might be mistaken. But to those who have worked around it, who have worked closely with the reaper on so many occasions, the lifeless human form is easily recognizable. To me, it's all in the eyelids. Keep your pupils. Even living pupils can be hard to read. But the eyelids tell the tale. Their pale translucence says that no blood flows through them. Their texture, like putty in death, is inanimate, a return to the clay of creation. It's as if the dead were once again a model of who they were born to be. But more, the way those lids move speaks volumes. If I open them when they are closed, it is as if they were closed on the sweetest of dreams. And if I close them when they were open, I imagine that they close sluggishly because the eyes they covered now gaze on sites indescribable and incomprehensible. I always go for the eyelids first. Then, I write my note, fill out the state form and return to the care of the living, who are much more difficult to read and never stop talking.

Most of those I have pronounced have been quite old. When I stand and look at them I see that we are all so fragile in the end. When life has left us, when the vibrancy that animates even the ancient has gone with the last breath, the shells that our bodies finally become seem pitiful, shattered porcelain jars, their contents spilled as their substantive parts evaporate into the universe.

 Still, mean as they appear I always consider how great is this last payment, this insight they give me as they slip away. So few people have seen death in these sterile times. If asked to pronounce someone dead, most would write it in their diaries as an event of stress and anxiety. But I have the gift of perspective, granted to me time and time again as a sort of last will and testament from all those I have touched after their departure. When I see them, I wonder about their lives and the events that shaped them. I marvel that each human is a library of stories, a warehouse of loves and hates. With every death we lose things that can never be recovered. That is the way it has always been. Only God remembers all.

More powerful still, this contact allows me a gift of meditation on my own demise. I realize that though I am young and the father of small children, there is no promise of tomorrow. And one of the forms of death that I have studied, or seen, cared for, struggled against, or finally surrendered a patient to, will be my own. Death visits mankind in many ways and there are quite a few I have not seen, but there is little new in the world. Will it be an MI? Will it be an infectious disease like pneumonia or sepsis? Or will I drive my car in front of a much larger one and go off to the crash of metal?   Maybe more interesting; in my old age I'll be eaten by a bear on a hunting trip in Alaska.   (Such deaths seem tragic, but one is remembered in family legend for years!).   Even better, hopefully my family will surround me as I slip away from who knows what, touched by my children, grandchildren and great-grandchildren.

So really, this pronouncing of the dead is far more than annoyance. It is wisdom in the making.   When my own patients die, I'm anxious.   I wonder if I did anything wrong.   I realize I have to face the family. And though I have many of the same emotions, it is not such an easy time of meditation.   But for these who were not my patients, who lie in well-made hospital beds, having fallen asleep from this life, I am grateful.   I am wiser, and more alive for every time that I certify "Date and Time of Death".

Doing Less is More

Like many professionals I have a long list of things to do. As a physician it includes such things as "read continuing medical education" and "discard stack of worthless mail". As a resident of rural Oconee County it includes "cut brush on property" and "find suitable location for tree-stand". It also says "write novel that changes course of history" and "spend time laughing with wife and children". However, I invariably get stuck on that last one. I suppose I need to enroll in a time management course; I'll add that to the list. The thing is, I simply can't look my family in the eyes and tell them I'm too busy. Consequently, my mail piles up, the brush grows tall and the book isn't published. But I can play a very good pirate (convincing to two toddlers at least). And I actually know my wife Jan's feelings by the flash of her blue eyes.

There are drawbacks to this lifestyle I have chosen. I will always have a certain haze of chaos in my life and thus accumulate mountains of untouched "to do" lists. It is unlikely that I will ever assume any political or academic position in medicine, because I have an allergy to meetings. And anything lengthy that I hope to write will probably take decades. But if that is the price, then I'll pay it. Because productivity is over-rated.

I'm speaking to the millions of people who feel continually driven. To those whose jobs offer them bonuses and promotions for just a little more sacrifice. Or those whose personalities require that they involve themselves in one more project or volunteer organization. Productivity is a modern addiction.

I've known some physicians whose jobs are their lives. Their homes are those places where they sleep and where their children learn the painful lesson of their relative importance. They attend soccer games by cell-phone and give a few sparse hours a week (scheduled ahead of time) to their sons and daughters. After this, they retreat to the computer to write that journal article until the wee hours, then rise again at 5am to run, shower, go to work and start again. Medicine being my field, I can't comment much on any other. But I know the same pattern of behavior exists in every other endeavor. There are always those who could do less, but can't stop.

The frantic life causes a deterioration of family. And in an age when we are rediscovering family values, time is the unmentioned but critical ingredient. Families aside, our maddening pace causes many to miss the joy of life. How often are we too busy to attend the rituals of our culture? The weddings, funerals and celebrations are portals into joy and sorrow, into the essence of our humanity. It is an unusual job or project that brings us that close to our fellow travelers. What about the simple pleasure of being alone? I think that the pace of our lives is sometimes intended to help avoid the agonizing clarity of being alone with our thoughts, just as the massive self help sections of bookstores are intended to fill in for the difficult tasks of self-examination and contemplation.

Productivity is important for everyone. We need to feel that we contribute positively to our jobs and communities; that we make a difference. But we need to remember that we need not reach exhaustion. And that the manner in which we influence those immediately around us, as well as the manner in which we seek our own well-being, is just as important as anything we do for strangers, corporations or governments.

Late last year my relative lack of productivity paid off. I discovered, in one small moment in time, that all my achievements and goals are as tangible as shadows and smoke while those things of real value are subtle, but solid as diamond. My oldest son, Samuel, had a third birthday party. The house was filled with screaming toddlers, wrapping paper, toys and a piñata. It was great fun and afterward, when the guests went home, Samuel and I had an errand to run. In the car, I asked him who, of all the guests, he enjoyed playing with the most. "You Papa", came the reply. We almost went that minute to buy a pony. What attainment could bring me the satisfaction of that moment? I hope I never find out.

Important Discharge Instructions

All too often, I discharge a patient and think to myself, "what instructions can I give for this?" Sometimes there are problems and questions, signs and symptoms that don't have very obvious solutions or answers. And in these situations, coming up with something useful for the patient to read at home is, to say the least, very difficult. So I've come up with a few based on some common night-time enigmas I see in my practice.

1) Virginity evaluation: The emergency physician has not determined the status of your daughter's virginity. In fact, the emergency physician does not wish to know the status of your daughter's virginity. Furthermore this doesn't really constitute an EMERGENCY. Unfortunately, no one has so far developed any simple home kits for making this determination. If you do, please notify the emergency department so that we can refer families to your product. If you wish to know more about your daughter's sexuality, try talking to her. If you found her naked in bed with a boy, it probably wasn't biology homework, no matter what she said.

2) Drug use evaluation: The emergency physician has not performed a random drug test on your teenage son, as you have requested so adamantly. He has no complaints, is not suicidal and has no apparent medical problem. This is not a family counseling center. If you want to know if he is using drugs, talk to him. Admittedly, he is a surly, unpleasant, disheveled and foul-mouthed young man, whose multiple piercings make him look like a Stone Age erector set. But finding out if he is or isn't using drugs simply doesn't constitute what we like to call an EMERGENCY. If he isn't using drugs, be certain that repeated trips to the emergency room accompanied by screaming parents will certainly give him good reason to start.

3) Whole body numbness: It simply isn't possible to be awake, walking, talking and functioning and be entirely numb from head to toe. Admittedly, your ability to overcome the sensation of sharp needles and other painful stimuli is impressive and may herald a future career with the CIA. For now, however, our physician has determined that the one thing likely to be numb on your person is your skull.

4) Pain Scale overview: We're sorry that you are in pain. We have attempted to fully evaluate your complaint and treat it appropriately. By now, we feel your pain also. But it is apparent that you don't fully understand the system we use called "the pain scale". Now, on a scale of 0 to 10, zero means no pain. This actually happens, believe it or not. Every day, millions of people wake up, work, go home, play and everything else without pain or the use of narcotics. It sounds spooky, we realize, but it happens. Ten, however, means the worst pain you can possibly imagine. Since this can be difficult to assess, here is a list of ten very painful things with which to compare your obviously impressive degree of suffering. A dental drill through the front tooth without anesthesia. Being eaten alive by an extremely hungry shark. Having your legs crushed under the wheels of a train. Being boiled in water or oil. Being dragged behind a truck through cactus while naked. Cutting half of the way through your leg with a chainsaw. Being hit in the face with the butt of a rifle by a well-seasoned Marine. Having your hand smashed by a sledgehammer. Breaking your leg so badly that the bone comes through the skin. Sparring with Mike Tyson. We hope this helps.

5) Alleged spider bite: In the summer, insects and spiders can be real trouble. Thank you for allowing us to evaluate the faint red mark on your body that you are convinced will prove fatal. The good news is, it won't! The bad news is, we can't tell you exactly what species caused it. It probably wasn't a spider. It certainly doesn't matter, since your only complaint is of said red mark. If you begin to show signs of dying in relation to this event, please return

immediately. Otherwise, remember that insect bites are seldom an EMERGENCY. And please wear a shirt from now on since this is a family hospital and your tattoos are for mature audiences only.

6) Fight with significant other: Please know that we understand your situation. Everyone has fights with spouses, boyfriends, girlfriends and all the rest. It's part of what we like to call life. It's unfortunate that your event was so earth shattering that it required an ambulance to bring you to the emergency department. But it has become evident that you suffered only emotional scars. You may have passed out, but in the good old days, doctors simply referred to this behavior as "hysterical", whether it involved a man or a woman. The bad news is that we have no control over your relationship and really have no interest in being involved in it unless you are actually injured by someone. If you look outside the hospital, you'll notice the striking absence of any sign that says "Jerry Springer Show". So please, take your drama somewhere else. The good news? Make-up sex is sometimes the best! And by the way, this doesn't constitute what we like to think of as an EMERGENCY!

7) Confused or weak nonagenarian with dementia: We appreciate the love that you obviously have for your family member. Thank you for trusting us to care for them. But just take a minute and ask yourself: "when I have dementia and I am 90 to 100 years old, can I expect to be weak or confused?" The answer, dear friend, is yes. So treat grandma or grandpa with love and respect, keep them happy and comfortable. But don't expect them to take up gymnastics or website development as hobbies.

8) Insomnia: The inability to sleep is very frustrating. We in the emergency department are familiar with this problem. In fact, we may be awake right now when we would prefer to be asleep. (We may also be asleep but appear to be awake). As frustrating as your insomnia is, two facts remain. It isn't an EMERGENCY and being in the hospital after midnight is not going to increase your chances

of slipping off to dreamland with your fantasy date. So run along and stare at the ceiling at home. If you go home now, one of the nurses will call you and sing a lullaby.

9) Get out of jail free card (i.e., officer, I can't go to jail because I'm too sick!). Thank you for the opportunity to evaluate you on the way to your incarceration. It makes us feel a part of the criminal justice system. Unfortunately, you have not exhibited any symptom that might keep you from your just rewards. If your complaint was chest pain, it isn't your heart or anything else dangerous. If your complaint was seizure, please practice more, as your attempt was substandard. If the police brought you here because you are intoxicated, we apologize. They obviously underestimated your capacity for surviving large amounts of alcohol. At any rate, you are good to go! Enjoy your well-deserved rest at public expense. Hopefully you'll learn your lesson this time.

10) "I think I have something I read about on the Internet:" The Internet is a wealth of knowledge. Your willingness to research your symptoms via computer is very self motivated. But remember, just because you read about it doesn't mean you have it. And just because it says that our physician should give you a particular drug for your supposed illness doesn't mean she or he will. After all, the computer can't actually see you or touch you. And the computer didn't go to medical school. We have examined you and we believe that you do not have the illness you are concerned about. So go back and surf the web if you like, but look at something more interesting than medical sites.

11) The emergency department menu: Your doctor may have suggested you need a powerful narcotic, or your friend may have told you that you need an antibiotic, but no one told us about it. You may have decided you need a prescription weight loss medication. Your wife may have told you to get some Viagra. (Ouch!). But the point is this emergency department doesn't have a menu. Don't look for it, because it isn't here. And the doctors and nurses aren't waiters. So

the bottom line is this: we aren't giving you what you want. And you didn't have anything approaching an EMERGENCY. The administration office opens at 8:30. You can lodge your complaint then.

12) "Nerves are shot": We're sorry that life is overwhelming. But since you don't appear to be a danger to yourself, or to anyone else, you're going to have to leave to make room for sick people. Hopefully, your anger at our department for failing to admit you for a much-needed rest will galvanize your will and give you something to live for. And to add to your anger, your life stresses are not actually an EMERGENCY.

13) Pre-litigation physical: Your motor vehicle accident sounds as if it was horrible. Having spoken to the paramedics, it is obvious from the lack of any damage to your car that all of the impact was transmitted through the frame of your vehicle, up into the upholstery of your seat, and directly to your neck and back. The problem is, this is not possible. You have not been injured. But cheer up, that hasn't stopped anyone else from getting a multi-million dollar settlement!

14) Work excuse: Boy, wouldn't we like to stay home from work because we partied too late! It's admirable of you to develop a bizarre and physically impossible series of medical complaints in order to obtain a work excuse. We respect your willingness to continue contributing to society by actually working. In fact, it puts you a notch above some of the folks we see whose main goal is avoiding work altogether. However, the answer is no. Several of us feel horrible today and a few actually had to care for sick, crying children all night before coming to work. But hey, here we are! Next time just be up front. "I'm here because I need a work excuse". You might actually get it! By the way, this wasn't really an EMERGENCY, was it?

A Jealous Mistress

I remember residency as the time during which I neglected my wife. We had dated for six years and were married just prior to the beginning of my training. She endured me as a pre-medical student and a medical student. I was driven, committed, focused and entirely self-absorbed. Still, she tolerated me knowing as she did that medicine was what I wanted. She, like so many good women, actually loved her husband more than he loved himself. So, after I finished all of the preliminaries, she must have believed that I would finally act like a husband having at last become the doctor I wanted to be. Poor girl, she was wrong.

Because once I was a resident, I was worse. In residency I began to believe I was as important as I had hoped to be before. In residency, I was at last in my place of professional and masculine bliss. I was a flight surgeon with an Air National Guard F-16 squadron. I was training in a trauma center, surrounded by the terrible accidents and diseases I so wanted to learn about. By my second year I was flying as a crewmember with the helicopter service run by the hospital where I trained. I was moon-lighting in local hospitals. I was making money. I was contemplating future careers. I was I.

Unfortunately, that was the heart of the problem. I wasn't part of the pair that my wife and I were supposed to make. She expected a husband but got a roommate. My wife was something other, the woman I loved but too often ignored. The woman I saw too seldom. The woman I spent too little time attending to.

Looking back on those days before children, I see that if I had been a real husband we could have enjoyed our lives much more. We could have traveled more than we did, we could have danced on our nights off, we could have taken more walks on the campus of the small college where she worked and we lived the first year. But we didn't, because I was too absorbed in myself and in medicine as a whole. That old saying about how medicine is "a jealous mistress" is true. But she's a cold mistress, a demanding one, who leaves you empty when you finally realize that that life exists outside of hospitals, in places where your first name isn't doctor and your last name isn't MD.

The thing is, physicians in training have a lot of excuses for their absences, physical and emotional. They use things like conference schedules, grand rounds, in-services, interesting patients, unique opportunities, drinks with friends and extra money moonlighting, all as justifications for what is, too often, their own lack of respect for the women or men whom they purport to love.

Unfortunately, these habits don't die when residency ends. The same self-aggrandizing behavior, the same cruel disregard follows them when they leave their residencies and go to other states, other towns and other hospitals. Eventually, it transforms quite nicely into disregard for their children, who are much less capable of rationalizing and much more capable of believing that their doctor parent doesn't really care much for them after all. Finally, this worship of medicine and self paves the way to the divorce court, where years spent together are simply butchered and the physical remains split between a man and woman who once were in love.

Happily, my marriage did survive. My wife saved it, or she and God saved it, working together to reach me and shake me back into the reality that I was not alone. I haven't forgotten the lesson. But many medical marriages perish.

So if I have anything to say to residents, it isn't about patient care, or politics; it isn't about contracts, insurance policies, malpractice or fee-schedules. It's that if they have someone they are supposed to love, they are not excused from it because they are in training. They are not excused from it because they are busy or tired, or because they are engaged in something intense and frightening. If they have someone they are supposed to love, it is their duty to love that person more than medicine, patients, excitement or self.

And while they are in training, they should train their hearts as well. They should have the discipline of true love, which puts their beloved first. They should, therefore, have a weekly date with their love, if only a date that involves eating carry out food in bed. They should listen to the one who loves them and who may be able to help solve their problems. They should develop genuine interest in the lives of their lovers, supporting them just as they want to be supported. And they must and I mean this, must consider their beloved in any significant

137

decision, especially those decisions like jobs after residency, that will deeply impact their partner's lives.

I wish that I could go back and be a husband to my wife, the kind I should have been. But I can only go forward, trying to love her better with the years we add to our lives. I just hope that residents everywhere, in every specialty, learn to love early and well. It will add years to their lives, years to their careers, lifetimes to their marriages and delight, sheer delight, to the hearts of those who care for them most of all.

Lost in the Wilderness of the Mind

"What kind of mother would I be if I left my son here and went home?" Reba asked me this with tears in her eyes. In the midst of a busy shift in the emergency room, it was a question I could not answer. Her son Jacob, in his twenties, was schizophrenic. He had wandered to our hospital over hundreds of miles. His mother thought he was dead, since he had been missing for months. The police notified her that he was in custody for some minor offense, so she came cross-country by bus and by taxi to our hospital in Seneca, South Carolina. She tried to pick Jacob up when he was released. He refused to go with her, but came to the hospital in a police car. I suppose he came to me because she asked him to, or because the police officers suggested it.

"He needs help," his mother said. "He needs to be committed and get help!" I talked to him. He was calm, not suicidal, not violent. I don't even think he was hallucinating. I spoke with the mental health counselor on call. South Carolina is a state with little money for mental health patients who are dangerous, much less those who aren't. The counselor said that Jacob didn't meet the criteria for hospitalization. He couldn't be forced to stay if he weren't an obvious danger to himself. There weren't enough beds for patients who were in peril, much less those who weren't.

I told his mother and she rolled her eyes, then fell back into her chair. "What am I supposed to do? I have to go back to work. I'll lose my job! I can't leave him here!" I tried to explain that I couldn't force him to stay. The law was just as rigid about that fact as anything else. "Well, he needs to get on the bus and go back home with me. That's it."

We discussed this with Jacob. He laughed and looked up and down. He stared into his hands. Every time that she asked him to go with her, he said no. She pleaded. She tried to speak gently. She tried to be rational. She tried to be firm. She cried.

In the end, we released him. I talked to her about outpatient mental health care. I was going through the motions. It was all pointless, really. Unless she could succeed. Unless he would get in the taxi that

139

we called, ride the 40 minutes to the bus station and go home with his mother.

The driver came. Reba begged her son over and over. She pulled on his arm. She tried to force him into the cab. She failed. There was nothing we could do. Physicians, nurses and deputies with years of experience intervening in lives and we were powerless. Jacob walked into the night with no money, no ID, no home and only the clothes on his back.

His mother shook with sobs as she left. She knew that it might be the last time she would ever see her baby. He would wander the land homeless and frequently confused. The next phone call might be the worst of all. Homeless schizophrenics get pneumonia, die of exposure, are murdered, walk in front of cars, develop HIV. The list goes on. His mother wasn't a physician, but she didn't need to be. She knew the score.

I've thought a lot about them since that night. I wonder if I'll see Jacob again. I wonder if he has moved on, east toward the coast or up to North Carolina. Maybe off to the labyrinth of Atlanta which, like New York City, could hide someone for a lifetime. I hope and pray he survives. For his sake and his mother's.

It all illustrates a difficult point in medicine and society at large. For all of our good intentions, we have limited capacity to fix lives. We can treat diseases. We can cure some of them. We can treat lives; we can cure very few.

At an unfortunate nexus of medicine, law and economics there is a blind spot, where some are simply outside of our collective reach. It's a reality that takes years to absorb, but it's the hard truth. Some people will just wander away no matter how much we want to help. And all we can do is whisper a prayer as they go.

Trailer Trash

We just moved to a new house. Somehow, over the last 9 years in our previous house, we accumulated an amount of material possessions that is actually greater than the combined volume of the old and new houses. It's some quirk of physics. Probably has to do with special relativity and fractal mathematics. Like I'd understand. Fortunately, there is a solution that is decidedly non-technological. The solution is the purge. The solution is to throw things away.

It sounds good but I'm very poor at it. The problem is not that I want to keep everything. Fact is, I want to have my new basement back. I need space to exercise. I need a room to store my arsenal. But since all of the stuff from the last house is stored there, only the act of throwing out trash will return my basement to me.

Over the years our accumulations have fallen into three categories. Things with emotional value, things with some potential use and things without either. The things without emotional connections or potential uses are easy. Give them away, sell them, burn them, I don't really care. The things that are useful I have difficulty trashing. A rug, a lawnmower someone could fix, some clothing no one wants. It's hard for me to consign things to the trash heap that might still serve some purpose. Some residual German utilitarianism from my ancestors. But the other things, that remind me of memorable times with Jan and the children, are a special problem for me.

You see, I can't bear to throw away toys that the children and I played with together, or that were special to them in ways adults can't grasp. I can't part with letters my wife and I have sent one another, or gifts we gave in love. I can't give away certain pieces of clothing that the children wore often and that I can still see them wearing in my mind's eye. The past clings to these items, somehow. So I'm hopelessly emotional about these things. And when I have a box to take to the dump that has even a faint hint of memory, I feel an almost physical pain.

I just can't refer to these things as trash. It's a word that I can't easily apply. That makes me either insightful, or a potential junk collector. I suppose "junk collector" is also in my genes. Like my uncle who collects vegetable boxes from the grocery store and stores them under the eaves of his house. Understandably, I hope it's insight.

Of course, trash is a word applied in other settings as well. I've heard it used in the emergency room on many occasions. It seems a particularly popular Southern description. "White trash,", "redneck trash", or the ever popular "trailer trash". It's typically used when patients with particular cultural connections are annoying, loud, demanding, drunk or addicted. Sometimes it's used when female patients carry themselves in, shall we say, "too forward a manner", with bright blue eye-shadow, high healed boots with mini-skirts, big hair and breast tattoos. For the gentlemen, it sometimes comes up when they are begging for more narcotics for their disability inducing back pain that became worse during a bar fight. They lie in blood stained t-shirts, mumbling into cell phones through broken teeth and swollen lips, trying to reach their mama or brother to come and get them. Sometimes, it seems like a word that fits.

But I've always had trouble with it. I'm not sanctimonious enough to lie and say I have never referred to anyone this way. I don't recall doing it to their faces, but sometimes I have behind their backs. Even when I have, however, it sticks in my throat. It makes my mouth dry. It gives me a vague sense of guilt. Because people just aren't trash.

They drive me crazy sometimes. I admit that I have a long list of unpleasant names that I mutter when I go from drunk to drunk in the middle of the night, smelling whisky scented vomit, sewing up lips and eyebrows, knowing if I miss anything I'll be sued by the drunk wretch, who will sit in court in a pressed suit acting like he intended to enter the priesthood until I ruined his life. I have my set of words for people who lie to me, who manipulate me, who rob me of the joy of my career. I have a vocabulary of late-night tirades for those who live from lawsuit to lawsuit, drama to drama, and for whom professional wrestling and Jerry Springer serve the same function as PBS in other families. But trash isn't part of that vocabulary, however unkind the other words might be.

I can't help but see each of them as someone's child, or someone's parent. I can't help but wonder if maybe they aren't very nice when the liquor wears off. I feel certain that a large number of them try their best, but just have weak moments and during those moments end up in my emergency room. They all have within them something useful, something that could help themselves and their fellow humans if only they could get to it, could strip away the surface and polish the heart, stretch the mind. Unfortunately, my experience leads me to think that this seldom happens. Because as the night shift doctor, I'm the team physician for Olympic class drunks, semi-pro street fighters, aspiring heroin addicts (Oxycontin will do just fine for now), and ladies who dance naked against metal poles on rickety stages in front of all of the above. They seldom change their paths in life. But hope always remains.

Oddly, I could call them trash if I hadn't talked to so many of them. I could call them trash if I didn't know a few of their stories, wasn't on a first name basis with them. I could call them trash if they didn't sometimes shake my hand and, through bruised eyelids and glassy eyes genuinely thank me for being there. I could call them trash if they weren't God's children.

I know I seem schizophrenic. I talk about the people I see like they're family, then I rant on and on about how these same people make me crazy. I always will. It's love/hate. They feel the same thing about me. We have an understanding. We have an uneasy truce. I'll do my best if they'll just show me a little respect. Neither of us expect miracles, so it works out OK.

My patients give me pleasure and pain. They give me insight and wisdom into the human animal. They scare me when I see what and who, lurks in the shadows of this life. But despite all of it, I can't bring myself to throw them out onto the dump. Because however they are, whoever they are, they still aren't trash. And it's precious few of them who are without any use. Most of them are a hidden combination of useful and valuable. And every single one of them has emotional value to someone. It may not be me. It may not be any other human on the planet. But God knows their names. And he never calls them trash.

143

Bobby, Jimmy and the big, honkin' snake

Two drunken buddies took a hike
one steamy summer day—
when suddenly they heard a noise
that took their breath away;

Said Bobby Dale, with slurry speech,
"I think I know that sound!"
And looking left and looking right,
he spied a rattler on the ground.

The two cried out with shear delight
and nearly wet their cutoff shorts,
cause messing round with rattlesnakes
was one of their most favorite sports.

Said Jimmy Joe, with blurry eyes,
"He's got a purty skin!
Let's smash his head and take him home
and make a belt of him!"

But Bobby Dale just shook his head,
and flashed a toothless smile,
"What's your rush old friend of mine,
let's have some fun a while!"

They dropped their six packs on the ground
to drink and have a sit,
and there to briefly ponder how
to keep from getting bit;

And Jimmy Joe looked up and said,
"I got a plan I think!
let's poke him with a stick, oh wait,
I need another drink,"

But Bobby Dale had bigger dreams,
"Whatcha' think of this?
How about I give that snake
a big ole' hug and kiss!"

Now Jimmy Joe was not that smart,
but smarter than his friend,
"Fun is fun you son of a gun,
but that might be your end!"

But Bobby's tattoo said, "ain't skeared"
so to the snake he shuffled
his flip flops slapping loudly left
his quiet cursing muffled.

And thinking he had seen it done
on television shows,
he bent right down and grabbed the snake
which promptly bit him on the nose.

Screaming out he threw it down,
then picked it up in anger;
the rattler had some more in store
and struck him on the wanger.

Lying down and screaming
he could feel the poison spread,
and Jimmy Joe ran up to try and
stomp the critter dead.

The snake too fast for barefoot Jimmy,
grabbed him on the thigh;
it held on tight as Jimmy prayed:
"Lord please don't let me die!"

The snake dropped off, his venom spent,
he wanted to get clear;
Bobby's face was swollen tight,
Jimmy left to find a beer.

And sitting down by Bobby,
whose throat was getting smaller,
he cracked that beer and sadly said,
"Don't matter if we holler,

Cause we're too far from anyone
for help to reach us here;
I reckon we'll just give it up,
at least we didn't showed no fear."

The coroner was quite confused
as he surveyed the scene;
Two pals with rigor mortis;
a snake in search of Listerine.

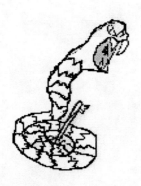

Fear

I wish that I knew the actual number of patients that I see each year whose symptoms, whether they know it or not, are actually a manifestation of anxiety. Sometimes it takes the form of chest pain. Sometimes, it appears as shortness of breath and hyperventilation. Occasionally, it presents as numbness or weakness, nausea or abdominal pain. And rarely, it leads a patient into a state of unresponsiveness, which friends and family believe is a coma, but in fact is simply a temporary time-out from life.

There are those persons afflicted with true anxiety disorders. Like the victims of any other disease, these people did not do anything to develop their illness. Their horrifying episodes of anxiety come at any place and any time and frequently for no reason whatsoever. But they are not the focus of my attention. For I believe that we live in a society eaten through with anxiety and filled with millions of persons who have had fear thrust upon them like some requirement for modern life, but which has robbed them of well being.

The truth is, although anxiety is responsible for a great deal of our unhappiness and ill feelings, it is also a powerful market tool. And, in some very odd way, it is an addictive drug to Americans. All one needs to do is turn on any investigative news show to find all of the things for which we are told, no one is worrying enough. As if our lives do not contain enough concerns, we are repeatedly told that we need more. This year, as the millennium approaches, the power of anxiety, the appeal of fear, is more manifest than it has perhaps ever been. If there is any message at the heart of the millennium, it is "live locally, worry globally".

The list is growing, but among the things deserving of our hand-wringing and sleepless nights are: Y2K, apocalypse, global warming, crime, SUV's, road rage, drought, famine, overpopulation, the rise of the Religious Right, the rise of the Humanistic Left, drug abuse, substandard schools, emerging infections, antibiotic resistance, planet killing asteroids, improperly cooked meat, urban sprawl, deforestation, nuclear war, biological weapons, cloning, violence in schools, violence at home, violence in the workplace, random violence, hate crimes, neo-

Nazism, gangs, militias, government intrusiveness, loss of privacy, the budget, Social Security, health care costs, civil litigation, etc., etc., etc. I suppose I could open any paper, read any newsmagazine or watch any network tonight and add quite a few new goblins to that ever-growing list. Is it really any surprise that our emergency department is so full of persons with anxiety? It's a wonder we leave home each day.

I have found myself a victim as well. Not long ago my wife Jan and I were taking a short trip and began to discuss our weekly events and concerns. She informed me, astutely as always, that I just needed to stop worrying. I suppose, in my mind, my defense was that bad things do happen. It's true. The world is full of causes for concern. Thus, I felt justified in my fears about my family having a car accident, about making a mistake in patient care, about the frightening turns that I believe the nation is taking and about not living up to my potential as a spouse, parent, physician, writer or anything else. (We all have a few custom made worries of our own).

She said that I just needed to stop. And I'm trying my best. Because I realized something critical. One of the reasons we pay attention to the calls of popular culture to worry is that we believe we can avoid something bad if we think about it. That it helps us to prepare for some eventuality. That somehow, fear is always how the universe says "Look out!" But the truth is, sometimes fear is just fear. A mind numbing, paralyzing, breath taking, chest crushing, life-sucking emotion that is, almost always, founded solidly in the imagination.

Fear is the devil's work. It robs us of more than our health. It robs us of the joy God created us to know. So, every night as I leave for work, I will continue to pray for God's grace, his undeserved protection. Because the alternative is the hopeless, constant, uncontrollable expectation of bad things. And life is just too short to live that way.

Crosses

When I drive, whether locally or to other parts of the country, I am always taken by the white crosses by the side of the road. Of course, they aren't always crosses. Sometimes they're wreaths, Stars of David, or Teddy Bears. Whatever they are, they interest me. They remind me, in a way, of historical markers. Like historical markers, they tell a story. I love stories. And even the sad ones have a place as they call us from our busy lives into the meanings of events outside ourselves.

When I was a child, trips to the cemetery were commonplace. I knew the appearance of the graves and headstones of many of my ancestors. My Grandmother and Grandfather Leap were buried in a cemetery high on a hill in the woods of West Virginia, overlooking a lake. The site is still vivid in my mind. It was a place of peace, not fear. And it was a place full of history and stories, some known, some unknown. There were gravestones from the early 1700's, some of them my own forebears. I remember walking in and out of the rows on Memorial Day and other times that we visited the dead. I remember marking the dates, the names, the ages and the inscriptions. There were some brought home from distant wars, some who died in accidents, some of age, some of epidemic. Each a complex saga only partially represented by the brief demographics carved in stone.

There was one large marker, designed to lie flat on the ground, which was broken in the middle for as long as I knew it. The inscription was weathered, worn and impossible to read. Local legend said that it was the burial place of a slave. I was always moved by this, imagining one who may well have come directly from Africa, to a land infinitely far away, unknown, to live, slave and die among those who were not his (or her) own. What an enormous tragedy to be buried among strangers and never have his or her story told, but lost to the ages except for folktales.

But every life is a story, really. Some lives are epic novels, some are short stories, concise and full of meaning. Some are even more brief and beautiful, like poems that speak volumes in a few short lines. Whatever the case, each life is worthy of being remembered and recognized, though few actually are.

The crosses that dot the highway force us to see that at that place, on some day we usually do not know, a story ended. The person represented likely started the day full of hopes and plans, expecting to go out and then return home. But the cross testifies to the fact that something awful interrupted those plans. Sadly, we can tell little more than the fact of the loss and an occasional name, as we speed by.

But even without the story; the crosses, stars, flowers and toys remind us that death is far more complex than television shows about trauma would indicate. Those shows give us the excitement of sirens and lights, the drama of the struggle with death. Sometimes they show the battle lost. But they never have the power of the markers by the side of the road. Because the markers remind us that a real person, who was loved and cherished, is now deeply missed. That when it occurred, someone received a horrible phone call or knock on the door from police with life shattering news. That family and friends will, for months, avoid that spot on the road whenever possible and will always see it as the place where they lost a part of themselves.

As the Upstate grows and our lives move faster, I believe the roadside markers serve the same function as cemeteries did in a slower and simpler time. They are drive-through reminders of our mortality. They force us to face the truth that news stories and statistics are comprised of unique, wonderful human lives.

I hope that changes can be made in road construction, vehicle safety and law enforcement that reduce highway deaths. But whether that happens or not, I'm going to take a few moments to think whenever I pass a marker. Maybe I'll be more careful and go a little slower. And hopefully, I'll reflect on one more story that I will never know and say a prayer for those who do.

The White Knights of Medicine

One morning last summer I went to a local ophthalmology office to have an assessment for refractive surgery (LASIK). I was the only patient in what would be considered a palatial facility by emergency department standards. The nurses and receptionists were all smiles. The floor was clean as a whistle. The marble counter tops sparkled. I filled out my tome of waivers and waited to be seen. I was escorted to the exam room by a very pleasant nurse who did tonometry, mapped my cornea and performed numerous exams that I probably wouldn't have understood if I'd read a book on them. I was seen by a very friendly ophthalmologist, with whom I had a great chat. I was pronounced a superior candidate, escorted back to the waiting room to speak to a scheduler, then given a can of soda and allowed to watch "Dances with Wolves" on the big screen TV in the waiting room (being too dilated to read). When my wife came to pick me up, I didn't want to leave. Wow. What a wonderful experience. But it was wonderful for more reasons than the courtesy that I received. It was a learning experience because it was a study in contrast to my own career.

My learning experience didn't have to do with improving my own customer service, or the cleanliness of my facility, or the smiles on our nurses' faces. It wasn't (although it crossed my mind) a learning experience about how my life might have been if I'd chosen a different specialty. It was, however, a profound insight into what a unique job emergency medicine is and about how proud we should all be.

I could have come away angry, given the cost of refractive surgery. But I wasn't. I could have been envious of the quiet environment and the nice furniture and sculpture. But my patients would just use sculpture to hold empty potato chip bags and cigarette packs. I did, however, come away disappointed in the way we treat our specialty and ourselves, for we are our own worst detractors and critics.

There are countless reasons that we emergency physicians should be impressed with ourselves. But mostly, they have to do with the things that conspire to make our practice of medicine difficult and which we somehow manage to overcome each day.

151

First, we practice in a specialty unlike any other, for we are self-proclaimed experts in an indefinable field of knowledge. Day in and day out, night after night we make snap decisions in two hours that would give most physicians hypertension and heartburn. We collate the half-truths presented as history with physical data that makes medical school look like fiction, then try to establish diagnoses in patients who often have problems that are far more social, psychiatric or purely imagined than physical. We deal with complaints that aren't found in any textbook, or we face medical nightmares so complex that all we can do is establish the ABC's and punt. We are a creative group of cowgirls and cowboys.

We also practice in an environment that is as close to a legal minefield as the metaphor will allow. In spite of our requirement to see patients for free, we always run the risk of multi-million dollar lawsuits as thanks for providing that free care. And even as lawsuits loom all around, we are counseled to cut costs by ordering less, admitting less and taking more risk. Furthermore, as if the contingency suits weren't bad enough, we have to face the growing specter of federal accusations of fraud for honest errors in a hopelessly complex system of billing codes.

Likewise, we are the victims of social engineering. Since the government can't actually provide free care to everyone (nothing actually being free anyway), they creatively found a way to make us do it via EMTALA. This must surely be one of the biggest unfunded mandates in history, in which we fundamentally work as slaves to the federal government. (To be compelled to work without compensation being the very essence of slavery). And it isn't just the government. Our comrades in the specialty are continually coming up with more ways that we should be the instruments of social intervention, whether it is via mandatory reporting of domestic violence, counseling our patients about substance abuse, or immunizing in the E.D. There simply aren't enough hours in a shift to do all this for the people who might conceivably benefit from it. Thus, we come to expect too much of our limited time and then are led to feel guilty about it.

And in the midst of the madness, we are constantly reminded to be aware of the "customer service" aspect of our specialty. However well the customer service model might work in the general marketplace, it fails when the service must be provided for free. Imagine how long any industry or small business would remain solvent if it were compelled to give its services or products with only the possibility of payment. What if a department store were forced to give everyone clothes (everyone needs clothes, right?) and were not allowed to ask for payment on the spot? What if a barber could bill for haircuts, but not ask for compensation at the time the service was provided? No other industry that I can think of is forced to work under such conditions.

Finally, we don't practice a specialty that promotes long life and well-being. We work odd, varying hours that disturb our sleep cycles. Not only are we awake in the wee hours of the night; we are awake and stressed. We eat poorly, drink too much caffeine and do too few things to promote our personal happiness. Furthermore, we are constantly exposed to the risk of communicable diseases or violence in our workplace. And every minute of every shift, anything imaginable can come through the door, whether on an ambulance stretcher or in the arms of a distraught parent. It may be an apneic child, it may be an exsanguinating gang member, it's all ours to sort through and try to save. When we fail, we have the equally horrific task of telling family members, then watching as they scream and slump to the floor.

As an unforgettable illustration, one terrible night this past summer, my partner and I cared for another of our partners who sustained a lethal head injury in an MVA on the way home from a shift. Could we close the doors, hang a wreath and mourn? Of course not, for the patients kept on coming. What can I say? Surreal doesn't begin to describe our job.

So I'm weary of criticism. I think we are amazing. I think we do incredible things in conditions that most practitioners would find simply unbearable. We work hard, we work fast, we try to be nice when we are being cursed, we endure the disdain of other specialties who consider us incompetent (except after 5pm), and through it all, we manage to actually care for the people who come to us. They aren't always nice and they don't always pay us, but most of the time they need us and sometimes they actually appreciate us. You see, we are the white knights of medicine.

That may sound a bit melodramatic, but we are the members of the medical community who always do the right thing no matter what. We do it because we were trained to, because we consider it honorable and because the law requires it. We are in battle day and night. We always get to do the things no one else wants to do, to the people no one else wants to care for, like lumbar punctures on AIDS patients, sexual assault exams, "pre-jail screenings" of drunk felons and psychiatric commitments after hours. This is our world; these are our people. And someone has to do it.

In the end, I love what I do. My schedule is reasonable. I have time off with my wife and children. I make a good living. I meet lots of people, some nice, some not so much. Some normal, some bizarre. I usually know what's going to be in the newspaper before it comes out. Sometimes I bond with sociopaths; sometimes I act like one myself. I perform interesting procedures and make fascinating diagnoses. I am constantly entertained by waves of mind-numbing human stupidity. I talk to the dying and I talk to their families. And even though it may not always be fair, no one gets turned away for lack of money, so I get to view the world of medicine from the moral high ground.

I ultimately had my LASIK in the beautiful office with the nice marble and smiling nurses. And I didn't complain. Everyone chooses his or her own path. I'm proud I chose mine. And I encourage all my sisters and brothers in the specialty to be proud, because we provide an invaluable service to society. We mustn't let anyone tell us otherwise. As a specialty, we should try a little harder to praise our fellow troops and take pride in our role. And we should learn more often to ignore the volumes of negative studies and articles that seem to tell us, month after month, how poorly we serve the public. But most of all, we should never let ourselves believe that what we do and the way we do it, is anything less than heroic.

Author Biography

Edwin Leap is a practicing emergency physician and writer. He lives and works in western South Carolina. He was raised in Huntington, West Virginia, graduated from Barboursville High School and Marshall University, and received his MD from West Virginia University. He is married to Jan Mahon Leap, of Madison, West Virginia. They have four children.

Printed in the United States
82015LV00002B/175-414

9 781591 136293